The CARPAL TUNNEL Helpbook

Self-Healing Alternatives
for Carpal Tunnel and
Other Repetitive Strain Injuries

Dr. Scott M. Fried

PERSEUS PUBLISHING
Cambridge, Massachusetts

Cataloging-in-Publication Data for this book is available from the Library of Congress.
ISBN 0-7382-0455-2

Perseus Publishing is a member of the Perseus Books Group.

Find us on the World Wide Web at http://www.perseuspublishing.com

Perseus Publishing books are available at special discounts for bulk purchases in the U.S. by corporations, institutions, and other organizations. For more information, please contact the Special Markets Department at the Perseus Books Group, 11 Cambridge Center, MA 02142; 617/252-5298.

Text design by Jane Raese
Set in 10 point Walbaum Book
Illustrations by Joanna Libonati of Ascension Design and Miguel Pirela-Cruz, M.D.

First printing
1 2 3 4 5 6 7 8 9 10–04 03 02 01

The Carpal Tunnel Helpbook

Other books by Scott M. Fried

Light at the End of the Carpal Tunnel:
A Guide to Understanding and Relief
from the Pain of Nerve Problems

This book is dedicated to my wife, Laura,
without whom the Upper Extremity Institute and I,
as the physician I am, would not exist.

As a nurse, mother, and loving wife she has taught me qualities
that no school of medicine or book could ever teach. The need to
be caring, loving, understanding, and compassionate while also
being firm and pure of task are what Laura has brought to me.
She is truly the selfless heart of our success, where she takes
little credit yet deserves much.

To you, Laura,
my best friend, wife, and love of my life,
I dedicate this book.
It is for you and our patients.

Contents

Acknowledgments

I would like to thank my friend and former chief of therapy at the Upper Extremity Institute, Valerie Romano, for her help in the initial writing and layout of this book. She took my early concepts and our program and put it into a basic document that became a template for this work. I didn't anticipate that her early efforts would lead to the countless hours I would spend building upon the work she did for me.

To my patients, whom I continue to praise as my greatest teachers: Thank you for motivating and showing me that our methods do indeed work. You have helped me to create a program that can heal people and help many avoid surgery.

To my clinical staff at the Upper Extremity Institute, thank you for your input and help in reviewing and contributing to the thoughts and ideas in this book. To my secretarial staff, thanks for making the words appear, sending faxes and e-mails, and putting up with the schedule changes and the stresses associated with various stages of the publishing process.

To my brother and best friend, Dr. Richard Fried, and Drs. Maureen Schreiber and Karen Sox, thanks for teaching me about biofeedback and the power of the human mind to overcome nerve disease and pain. Also, thank you for your help in developing one of the first biofeedback programs in the country dedicated to the treatment of nerve pain and injury.

A special thanks to Dr. James Hunter, who years ago conceived the fact that physical and occupational therapy can be the best way to treat nerve disease and that patient education is the key to a happy patient and outcome. His vision and the basic premise for the motion and stretching process presented in this book have been my guiding principles. Thanks also to Lee Osterman and Bill Bora, who gave me my first exposure to hand surgery and continue to be my teachers and friends.

I also thank my good friend Frank Murphy for his legal and literary expertise in helping to prepare the initial text and especially for his thoughts on patient advocacy issues.

Thanks also to Nancy Henderson for her editing assistance. Her tactful but authoritative style in helping to refine this text can only be appreciated by those who have experienced the true editing process. If it can be called fun, Nancy made it so.

My agent, Gail Ross, is a special person. She and Jenna Land, her talented assistant, took on this project with finesse and charm and found the opportunity to work with the wonderful people at Perseus Publishing, including Marnie Cochran. Marnie has allowed me to take my dream of helping millions avoid pain and bring it to the public, skillfully navigating the course without deviation.

My wife, Laura, and our children, Josh, Allison, and Hannah, must be thanked, not because they are the light of my life and know more about carpal tunnel problems than they care to admit, nor because they have been there for me throughout the writing process in every way, nor because they help to edit my thought processes by lovingly criticizing my writing and lectures as I have formulated my own ideas. I thank them in truth for sharing their time, in allowing me to chase windmills and pursue a writing career, because they know it is in my heart and they love me enough to allow the time to make it happen.

Last, but not least, I want to thank my mom and dad. Having been born to a family of healers, it seems natural that I would pursue a similar direction. My parents taught me early on to love and learn from everyone. Mom taught me that all people are special and to see the good in all things, and she gave me my basic optimistic and happy outlook on life. She also showed me what a powerful force love and family can be.

My father passed away last year, but he still stays with me. All of those whose lives he touched, as a psychologist and as a human being, benefited from having known him. He taught me that although I am trained as a surgeon, my job is to take care of people and to understand them. He rightly pointed out that although there are many rewarding things a person can do with his or her life, few are as rewarding as the opportunity I have been afforded–to make a difference in people's lives, and to know that every day someone whose life I have touched will be happier and experience less pain because of what I have written.

Introduction

Over the years I have had the opportunity to treat thousands of patients with upper extremity nerve problems, which can involve the neck, shoulders, arms, wrists, or hands. These problems can result from traumas, sports, motor vehicle accidents, or, in many cases, repetitive motion or repetitive strain injuries. The latter often occur from jobs that require the use of computers, power tools, hand tools, or scanners, or from production line work.

Carpal tunnel "syndrome" has long been considered a surgical disease, but patients are gaining enough awareness to be able to trust their own judgment more than "conventional medical wisdom." The reality is that carpal tunnel problems, repetitive strain injury, and thoracic outlet syndrome are indeed NOT surgical diseases. Rather, they are problems that very often have simpler, safer, less painful, and more predictable treatments. With common sense and a realistic understanding of the underlying pathology of these injuries, nonsurgical treatment, including self-treatment, becomes not only achievable but also preferable.

Over the past twenty years, our understanding of nerve problems has come a long way. We now realize that nerve injuries are much more complex than simple "compressions" and "carpal tunnel problems." The idea that all upper extremity nerve problems are carpal tunnel is far outdated.

Those of us who work primarily with nerve problems in the neck, shoulders, arms, wrists, and hands have come to realize today that most patients with longstanding carpal tunnel problems have multilevel nerve involvement, not just local involvement at the wrist. We have been forced to remember that the nerves at the carpal tunnel begin at the neck, then travel down through the thoracic outlet and the arm and into the wrist and hand. Injuries can occur at one or more levels and need to be addressed accordingly. Furthermore, if the entire arm and upper body nervous system are not mobilized in the treatment process, then secondary sites of nerve fixation and involvement may develop or become symptomatic.

I have set out to present a basic compilation of our understanding of these nerve problems and simple treatment methods. Physicians, therapists, chiropractors, holistic healers, and other alternative and integrative healing professionals can also apply these methods. Even more important, patients can use this information on their own. With appropriate education, you as a patient can help treat yourself and avoid progressive problems and injuries.

This guide is not intended to be a replacement for professional diagnosis and therapy. Rather, it should be an adjunct to appropriate treatments performed under professional care and a handbook for patients.

1.

Nerve Problems in the Neck, Shoulders, Arms, and Hands

Amy was a 28-year-old graphics designer for a sweater manufacturer. She spent most of her ten-hour work day sitting on a stool, leaning over a flat table, drawing designs by hand. She was under considerable pressure to produce as many designs as possible each day.

The strain to maintain a speedy work pace was physically and mentally draining for Amy. Her right arm often fell asleep as she worked, and at night she awakened regularly with pain, numbness, and discomfort. For seven years she endured the pain, until the numbness eventually turned into a shocking sensation shooting through her arm. Her symptoms did not fit the typical picture of carpal tunnel syndrome, and when she consulted various doctors, none of them looked beyond her hands for possible injury in the neck area or other levels of nerve involvement.

Despite Amy's continued complaints of numbness, tingling, arm and neck pain, and headaches, which are all classic symptoms of repetitive strain injury, she was referred to a therapy program for strengthening her hand muscles and endurance training. Rather than improving, her symptoms gradually worsened, and her family practitioner referred her to me at the Upper Extremity Institute for further evaluation and treatment.

At our first meeting, Amy was haggard, depressed, and in severe pain. Electrical nerve studies called EMG/NCV confirmed that she had a carpal tunnel problem as well as thoracic outlet injury. We talked extensively about the repetitive arm and hand activities required in her work and the neck strain associated with her symptoms. Her health insurer and employer insisted that Amy's symptoms were not caused by her work. In many cases, patients are able to heal by modifying their work and other activities, but this was not an option for Amy. I told her that as long as she continued under her daily work pressures, she would not heal.

For most of her life, Amy had done as she was told and played by the rules. Instead of pursuing her secret ambition to become an actress, she had followed her parents' desire that she pursue a more conventional career. As she grew increasingly depressed by her situation, Amy's pain, disability, and inability to function physically and mentally became overwhelming. The physical discomfort was probably a factor in her difficulty with personal relationships as well.

During my first visit with Amy, we talked about the fact that she was very uncomfortable with the prospect of surgery and did not believe that it would cure her. When I suggested that a nonsurgical course could be more successful, we discussed the concept of integrative medicine and the possibility of modifying her lifestyle.

As Amy began learning more about her nerve injuries, she started to imagine how she might change her daily activities and her career. She benefited from hot packs, ultrasound, and other forms of therapy, as well as from nutritional supplements, including B-complex vitamins and antioxidants such as vitamins C and E. She enrolled in a yoga class and also began to use meditation, biofeedback, and other integrative healing techniques.

The transformation in Amy's life was wonderful to witness. She began to have more fulfilling personal relationships and to feel much happier and in better control of her life. This is not to say that her life was easy. She still had some pain, but she had become much better able to control it. When difficulties with romantic relationships set her back a couple of times, she managed to overcome her tough experiences and grow from them. Eventually, she formed a stable, loving relationship and began to pursue a new career as an actress as well as a new sales career in the nutritional products industry. At first her finances were a little tight, but soon she reached, and eventually surpassed, her previous financial status. She had overcome abuse of her body and had made optimal use of her other talents and personal assets.

Everyone has within himself or herself an innate capacity to heal. A crucial role of physicians and therapists who focus on upper extremity nerve injuries is to help people with carpal tunnel and nerve injury symptoms to unlock this self-healing capacity.

CARPAL TUNNEL:
AN EVOLVING PROBLEM

In the first half of the twentieth century, doctors were aware that many of the nerve problems they treated began in the neck area.

In the mid-1950s, Dr. George Phalen coined the term "carpal tunnel syndrome" for a nerve injury in the hand and wrist that had become common among elderly people with low activity levels who had worked hard for many years. Because these patients had sedentary lifestyles in their later years and often died at relatively young ages, surgery usually provided adequate pain relief. Dr. Phalen did not envision the complexities that would evolve as technology began to change the workplace. Eventually, "carpal tunnel syndrome" incorrectly became the common medical term for a variety of nerve problems in the upper extremities, including the neck, shoulders, arms, and hands.

Research in the 1950s and 1960s helped bring further understanding of the relationship between traumas sustained in daily life and nerve injury at the neck and lower arm. Exposure to vibration and repetitive stress from activities such as chicken boning and cleaving in the meat industry became well-known causes of nerve injury in the arms.

New types of injuries to the hands and arms became common by the 1970s, thanks to lifestyle changes such as increased use of computer keyboards, scanners in grocery stores, jackhammers, and three-point seatbelts in automobiles. Although they help save lives by holding the upper body in place, the new seatbelts also increase the severity of whiplash injuries.

Physicians eventually came to realize that many people are not cut out to posture their necks and arms at a computer all day, and they identified the computer keyboard and mouse as risk factors for injury to the hands and neck. Increasingly, they identified problems such as repetitive strain injury, carpal tunnel syndrome, thoracic outlet syndrome, fibromyalgia, and pain syndromes such as reflex sympathetic dystrophy, and often treated them with surgery.

By 1995, more than 500,000 surgeries for carpal tunnel and related problems were being performed annually in the United States, but many patients were failing to improve. Meanwhile, millions more began suffering from the pain of nerve injury in the hand, wrist, elbow, or neck but did not seek treatment.

Although surgery can be somewhat helpful, physicians and patients often have unrealistic expectations. A patient who returns to a job requiring full-time keyboarding or using a jackhammer all day is often doomed to failure. Understanding the causes of injury and the effects of work activities are essential to the healing process.

It has become apparent to me and to many of my colleagues that the medical community needs to be more aggressive in educating the public about nerve disease. In fact there is still confusion and misunderstanding among physicians pertaining to treatment of many of the problems discussed in this book. What we do know is that through better patient understanding and improved awareness of these problems, many patients are able to avoid surgery and lead normal lives through conservative care, such as therapy and modifying their lifestyles and activities.

Essential to treating any upper extremity nerve pain is learning how to take care of one's own body. Judicious use of deep heat, ice, ultrasound, high-voltage galvanic stimulation, and other therapies often relieves acute inflammation. Ancillary techniques such as biofeedback, massage, tai chi, and yoga provide relaxation conditioning. Nerve sliding, acupuncture, and visualization techniques help to decrease muscle spasm and can be extremely useful in decreasing nerve pain and even reversing the scarring process. These types of treatments help patients to be the essential ingredient and governor of their own healing process.

WHAT ARE CARPAL TUNNEL NERVE INJURY, THORACIC OUTLET SYNDROME, FIBROMYALGIA, AND REPETITIVE STRAIN INJURY?

CARPAL TUNNEL NERVE INJURY

The carpal tunnel is an area where the bones of the wrist come together in the shape of a shallow valley that is closed on the palm side

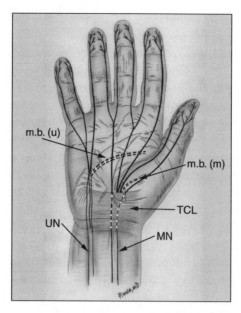

FIGURE 1.1   The Carpal Tunnel. The transverse carpal ligament (TCL) is
on the right, above the median nerve (MN); the ulnar nerve (UN) is at left.
The motor branch median nerve, m.b.(m), and motor branch ulnar nerve,
m.b.(u), are also shown.

by a band of tissue called the transverse carpal ligament (see Figure
1.1). Passing through this tunnel of bone and ligament are nine tendons and the median nerve. These tendons begin in the forearm muscles that help move the fingers. Each tendon is about the size and
consistency of a thick piece of linguine. The median nerve is about
the size of a pencil and has a smooth surface. The roof of the tunnel is
a tough strap of ligament.

Inflammation within this closed tunnel at the wrist is the underlying condition that leads to carpal tunnel problems. The tendons that
slide through the tunnel are surrounded and encased in a lining
called tenosynovium, which is a very thin substance that makes the
tendons slippery enough to slide easily through the carpal tunnel.
When the fingers move rapidly and regularly and the wrist bends up
and down, friction from the sliding tendons causes swelling. With
continued swelling, the synovium can thicken, taking up more space
than allotted in this tight tunnel. The decreased space results in in-

creased pressure on the nerve in the carpal tunnel, which can lead to numbness, tingling, pain, and discomfort.

A common cause of carpal tunnel problems is performing the same movements repeatedly for hours at a time. Carpal tunnel problems are sometimes accompanied by other diseases or conditions, such as arthritis, bone fractures, diabetes, or thyroid disease. As the inflammation underlying carpal tunnel injury worsens, it leads to scarring, and it binds the nerve down so that it will not slide, so it becomes chronically compressed. If this process continues, the patient develops a permanent, irreversible condition. As more scar develops around the nerve, less trauma or irritation is required to bring about the symptoms of numbness, pain, and dysfunction.

Early diagnosis, treatment, and conservative care are therefore vital. If left untreated, carpal tunnel problems may result in permanent injury and loss of the productive use of the hand. A physician or therapist can diagnose carpal tunnel involvement through a detailed history and physical examination, and with electromyelography and nerve conduction velocity (EMG/NCV) testing.

Symptoms of carpal tunnel injury may include:

- Numbness and or tingling in the fingers or hands
- Weakness or clumsiness in the fingers or hands
- Pain from the wrist that may seem to shoot up into the arm or down into the hand
- Pain or discomfort radiating or shooting up to the neck or down from the neck to the fingertips
- Burning in the fingers or hands
- Numbness or tingling, often on awakening from sleep

Generalized weakness and numbness can also be a sign of other disorders. Carpal tunnel nerve injury usually follows a specific nerve and pain distribution. For an accurate diagnosis, it is important that you, as a patient, be specific in telling your doctor where the pain is. Remember, not all doctors are great communicators, and your input and ability to relay accurate information is vital in obtaining a correct diagnosis. If your thumb and index finger go numb, be sure to say so. If you simply say "my hand or my arm," an incorrect diagnosis could result.

THORACIC OUTLET SYNDROME

The thoracic outlet is the triangular channel through which the nerves and vessels of the arm leave the neck. It is bounded by the anterior scalene muscle in the front, the middle scalene muscle in the back, and the first rib below. It is the tunnel or channel through which all of the nerves and blood supply travel into the arm (see Figure 1.2). In thoracic outlet syndrome (TOS), the nerves and sometimes the blood vessels that supply the arm are being irritated or compressed in this triangular area between the neck and shoulder. The irritation is usually caused by compression or scarring from tightness or injury in the muscle, bone, or ligament bands. Along with major arteries and veins, the nerve complex known as the brachial plexus is located in the thoracic outlet. It is the group of nerves that slide and move between the muscles of the neck and shoulder.

The brachial plexus nerve complex is a frequently overlooked component of our anatomy in investigations of possible nerve injury. In

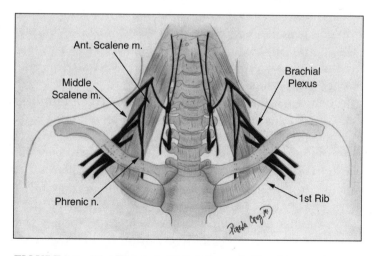

FIGURE 1.2   The Thoracic Outlet (bounded by the anterior scalene muscle in the front, the middle scalene muscle in the back, and the first rib below)

many cases, however, it is the actual cause of nerve pain and disability in patients who fail to respond to nonsurgical treatment, such as physical and occupational therapy, splints, and nonsteroidal anti-inflammatory or pain medication. Many patients who "fail" at surgery for carpal tunnel or repetitive strain injuries actually have thoracic outlet or brachial plexus injury that has gone unrecognized.

The brachial plexus nerves travel through the tunnel or space of the thoracic outlet and form all of the nerves that go into the arms and hands. The nerves in our arms and legs are capable of sliding and bending between tissues, thus allowing us to move without harming them under normal conditions. When this sliding does not occur easily, or when there is direct pressure on these nerves, pain and nerve symptoms develop.

Compression of the plexus or scarring of its nerves can result from many sources, both internal and external to the body. Repetitive upper extremity activities and prolonged stress-inducing positioning, such as chronic neck flexion, are major sources of compression and nerve scarring. Certain abnormal postures, shoulder movements, and poor breathing habits can aggravate symptoms by pulling on the nerves and narrowing the thoracic outlet.

Thoracic outlet injury can result from compressive, neurogenic (nerve scarring), or, in rare cases, vascular (circulatory) causes. Injury from compression may come from the presence of an extra (cervical) rib or from injury to the scalene muscle. The vast majority of injuries have neurogenic causes and involve scarring about the nerves and compression.

Researchers and clinicians believe that TOS has a number of different causes. The earliest reports on TOS centered on the presence of bony abnormalities such as an extra rib in the neck with circulation abnormalities, but it turns out that fewer than 10 percent of patients with TOS have this abnormality. Trauma is often the precipitating factor in the development of TOS. What we may think to be minor trauma, such as repetitive motion of the arm, may cause changes in the tissues around the nerves and the scalene musculature. Activities such as repeatedly reaching (using a grocery store scanner, for example), extensive typing, or regular use of a computer mouse can result in increasing irritation of the tissues about the thoracic outlet and the wrist. This scarring about the nerves and narrowing of the thoracic outlet compromises the ability of the nerves to travel or slide freely.

Injury to the nerves of the brachial plexus often results from whiplash-type injuries in car accidents, caused by sudden deceleration and rebound acceleration. Such injuries may also come from activities that require looking up or down in abnormal ways or repeatedly kinking or straining the neck.

Forceful side-bending injuries of the neck may result in tearing of the scalene muscle, even at a microscopic level, or yanking or ripping of the fine, cobweblike supporting scar tissue (fascia) that holds the nerves of the brachial plexus in place. When this tissue about the nerves is torn or the muscle itself around the nerves is injured, inflammation results. A thicker adherent tissue may form and bind down the nerves of the plexus, resulting in pain, discomfort, and disability.

Brachial plexus problems may occur in very subtle ways from repetitive minor traumas, such as repeatedly reaching–as waitresses do–using a jackhammer, or even using a regular hammer. Yanking or pulling injuries on the arm may also result in tearing of these tissues. Prolonged abnormal posturing of the neck and shoulders is a much more subtle yet common mechanism for the development of brachial plexus or thoracic outlet injury.

Continued strain on the soft tissues results in chronic inflammation and subsequent scarring, restricting the nerves and their blood supply. This is a significant problem for people who sit at a computer keyboard for long periods, especially in poorly designed work environments. Holding a telephone receiver on the shoulder or with the arm bent can cause chronic "kinking" of the neck as well, which is also a form of injury to the thoracic outlet. Direct blows to the shoulder or plexus area can result in similar injuries.

Injuries can be further complicated by the fact that the sympathetic nerves enter the arm through the nerve of "Kuhns" at the lower trunk of the brachial plexus. Many patients with thoracic outlet or brachial plexus problems therefore exhibit other symptoms that do not fit classic nerve distributions and clinical pictures. Problems such as color changes in the hand, swelling, and variations in temperature of the hand or arm are often confused with reflex sympathetic dystrophy (pain syndrome) or interpreted as overreaction to pain.

FIBROMYALGIA

Fibromyalgia, or fibromyalgia syndrome (FMS), is a diagnosis carried by millions of Americans today. It is a poorly defined disease, hallmarked by the presence of general symptoms such as pain, swelling, fatigue, aches of a very generalized nature, sleep disturbance, and, often, depression. Patients generally have significant difficulty with lack of energy and an increased amount of aching or pain with activity and exposure to minor injury. They are more likely to have inflammation or joint swelling than the general population when exposed to minor traumas in daily living. For example, simply typing a letter could cause significant pain that lasts for a day or longer.

Fibromyalgia appears to be a low-level form of arthritis, in which standard blood tests are negative for more easily classified conditions, such as rheumatoid arthritis and lupus. It is classically accompanied by the presence of diagnostic trigger or tender points elicited by pressure in specific areas.

Interestingly, many of these trigger points are in the upper back and arms, and they correspond directly with the path and distribution of the nerves commonly involved in thoracic outlet syndrome and repetitive strain injury. Specifically, the long thoracic nerve in the upper back between the spine and scapula, the posterior occipital nerve in the back of the head, and the radial nerve in the forearm are involved.

Many of the other symptoms, such as sleep disturbance, fatigue, and pain that changes in intensity and distribution, are also found in patients with nerve injury such as thoracic outlet syndrome and repetitive strain injury.

Fibromyalgia generally does not involve joint deformity or other telltale diagnostic evidence, so patients are often undertreated. Reflex sympathetic dystrophy in its less severe form may have many of the same symptoms as fibromyalgia. In fact, many patients have fibromyalgia as well as nerve disease. Often, one accompanies the other in presentation, and repeated injuries may indeed lead to a chronic inflammatory state that is responsible for the onset of all of these pathologies.

Treatment that emphasizes lifestyle modification, appropriate use of exercise and medications, meditation, and relaxation techniques is quite effective in treating fibromyalgia as well as nerve injury.

REPETITIVE STRAIN INJURY AND DOUBLE-CRUSH SYNDROMES

Thoracic outlet syndrome, carpal tunnel injury, and repetitive strain injury often have similar symptoms, which can confuse physicians, therapists, and healers and lead to incorrect diagnoses or ineffective treatment. When injury occurs in two places, such as the neck and the wrist, the result is sometimes called a double-crush syndrome.

Imagine that you are in your yard on a bright sunny day, watering your garden with a hose. Your neighbor comes along and initiates a conversation. Inadvertently, she stands on the hose. You may not notice any significant change in the flow of water because the amount of pressure on the hose is relatively small. This is similar to a low-level nerve problem with no obvious symptoms (see Figure 1.3).

While you are conversing with your neighbor, her husband arrives and joins in the conversation. Unfortunately, he too stands on the hose, a few feet down the line. Suddenly you realize there is not enough flow to water your plants. Your neighbors have compromised the flow in the hose, creating a double-crush type of problem. Your nerves are like the hose. With pressure in two places, the flow of

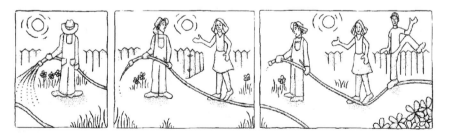

FIGURE 1.3   Double-crush Syndrome Can Be Likened to a Garden Hose Being Stepped on in Two Places

nerve impulses has been reduced or slowed enough for you to feel symptoms.

If a garden hose were pulled and stretched with enough force, it would narrow and decrease water flow like a traction-type nerve injury. This phenomenon also causes decreased flow of impulses and can cause one or more levels of poor flow. It can be likened to a stretch injury to the brachial plexus and can result in a second level of nerve injury, or double crush, especially if there is a preexisting asymptomatic carpal tunnel problem.

Double-crush involvement usually occurs by the neck and near the elbow or the wrist and hand. The overall flow and speed of electrical conduction can slow to the point at which the brain interprets a significant delay in impulse conduction. This results in numbness, pain, tingling, or weakness. Unfortunately, patients suffering from this phenomenon are often labeled with incomplete diagnoses. If some of their symptoms remain after carpal tunnel surgery, they may be categorized as "treatment failures."

Because the nerves begin at the neck and travel as long structures or cables through the arm to the fingertips, injury can occur anywhere along this circuit. Scarring, inflammation, or compression at the thoracic outlet, at a disc at the neck, at the ulnar or radial nerve by the elbow, or in the carpal tunnel median nerve at the wrist can all produce nerve symptoms. Pathology at the thoracic outlet often accompanies other nerve symptoms. In fact, most thoracic outlet and repetitive strain injuries involve multiple levels of nerves.

Because of complexities in the brain's ability to process nerve information, it often seems impossible for a patient or physician to tell exactly where nerve entrapment has occurred, especially when more than one set (or level) of nerves is involved. This makes it particularly important that doctors, therapists, and other healing professionals listen very carefully to a patient's complaints.

When a practitioner listens carefully and provides a comfortable environment, a patient can almost always describe and define the symptoms of a thoracic outlet or brachial plexus problem, a carpal tunnel entrapment, a repetitive strain injury, or local involvement of a nerve at the elbow. Patients with thoracic outlet problems regularly complain of symptoms that involve activities such as reaching, pulling, pushing, or lifting overhead. Activities such as combing or blow drying the hair can be very difficult and can cause the arms to go numb. Many patients even rearrange their kitchens so that dishes are on lower shelves. They often have pain and discomfort at night, which may involve awakening with numbness or lying on the involved side or with an arm overhead. Driving is often problematic for these patients because of their posturing of the head, neck, and arms.

Patients with thoracic outlet and repetitive strain injuries often give a history of progressive problems that evolve over time and result from minor traumas or motions repeated time after time. Patients often relate that their hands or wrists initially bothered them and a well-meaning friend or physician gave them splints. They continue to perform repetitive activities, but because the splint does not allow wrist motion, they begin using their elbows repetitively and posture their arms in an abnormal manner. Over the course of time, the elbows became uncomfortable, and problems develop at the radial tunnel or lateral epicondyle, such as tennis elbow. Then, trying not to move their elbows too much, they start overusing the shoulder. Excessive reaching and gross whole-arm movements substitute for finer dexterous lower arm use, and they perform simple activities in an awkward posture to compensate for the pain.

At this point, the nerves are being yanked and pulled at the level of the brachial plexus as well as the lower arm, and the problem becomes unlivable. Progressive inflammation occurs, along with swelling and scarring about these nerves. Ultimately these patients develop full-blown repetitive strain injury, thoracic outlet syndrome, carpal tunnel, or ulnar nerve problems.

If the insults continue, the scarring at all levels becomes a significant problem that is not likely to be reversed. Once a person reaches this point, a fixed nerve injury is present and will likely require surgery. That is why it is so important that employers and employees become aware of this sequence of events and how to recognize and address them early on.

Doctors and patients working together can avoid the development of a full-blown thoracic outlet problem and repetitive strain injury and even help reverse the symptoms. When patients learn how to modify their lifestyles and activities, they are often able to obtain symptom relief.

OTHER SYMPTOMS

Many patients, especially those who have involvement at the neck or thoracic outlet level, exhibit symptoms that are not usually associated with peripheral nerve injury. These symptoms are often the result of involvement of the sympathetic nervous system and the cervical plexus, and they may range from color changes in the hands and arms to painful burning sensations in the chest or upper back.

It is not uncommon for a patient with a thoracic outlet problem to describe stabbing pain in the chest, which is often associated with the anterior axillary nerve in the chest wall. Upper back pain, between the spine and scapula, is often associated with involvement of the long thoracic nerve, which travels down the upper back between the spine and the scapula or wing bone.

Pain can even radiate into the face, ear, or eye. Headaches are common, coming from the base of the skull, emanating from the posterior occipital nerve. Some patients report blurring of vision, ringing in their ears, or hearing changes. Temporo-mandibular joint symptomotology (TMJ) is also frequently associated with upper extremity nerve problems. Repetitive strain injury and fibromyalgia sufferers often experience involvement of the nerves of the brachial plexus.

Although the odds may be high that seemingly unrelated symptoms you experience are related to your nerve injury, it is important to have heart symptoms checked out by a heart doctor, breast complaints by your gynecologist or family doctor, and ear or facial symptoms checked out by the appropriate ear, nose, and throat specialist.

On more than one occasion I have sent patients with substantial nerve symptoms accompanied by chest pain for an evaluation by a cardiologist, who then found an underlying cardiac problem along with the nerve injuries.

NERVE HEALING

The nerves have a wonderful innate capacity to heal themselves. Given the proper environment and appropriate treatment, many nerve problems will calm down and actually reverse their damage. It is only when nerve inflammation and swelling reach the point of significant scarring, compression, and inability to slide or move normally in the tissues that nerve problems become fixed or permanent and require surgical intervention. Once symptoms require surgery, the expectation for recovery and return to full function becomes much less predictable. This is why early diagnosis and lifestyle modification are crucial.

Thoracic outlet syndrome and repetitive strain injury have existed for many years. The very nature of these problems helps explain many of the signs and symptoms present in patients who do not exhibit the classic patterns of commonly seen lower arm nerve injury problems.

Although some patients may be predisposed to developing thoracic outlet syndrome, repetitive strain injury, and carpal tunnel problems, there is usually an identifiable underlying cause especially if the problem becomes predominant to the point of severe symptoms and disability. With certain injuries or cumulative minor insults, increased tension and friction on the muscles, nerves, and tendon structures subsequently leads to progressive compression or traction patterns. The resulting inflammation produces exudate (fluid), which results in swelling and can eventually solidify into fixed scar tissue.

Round-shouldered postures or working in a poor ergonomic environment may predispose patients toward nerve injury. Some patients' poor postures may involve an effort to adjust their position to help decrease the pull on scarred or compressed nerves. I often observe patients holding the involved shoulder up closer to the ear to decrease the pull on the brachial plexus nerves.

A doctor may order a diagnostic work-up to confirm the presence of thoracic outlet syndrome. MRI scans and X-rays may show bone or disc abnormalities in the neck or chest or the presence of an extra cervical rib. They also help rule out conditions such as fractures and arthritis. Electrodiagnostic tests or nerve studies, such as EMG/NCV studies and somatosensory evoked potentials (SSEP) testing may help confirm a diagnosis by measuring the speed at which the nerve can conduct electrical impulses.

Be aware, though, that a negative test does not mean you don't have a problem. It may be that it is either too early to show changes or that the test or examiner was not able to identify the pathology.

As a patient, your best bet for symptom relief is to receive a thorough explanation of your individual problem and to try options such as behavior modification, relaxation techniques with biofeedback, supervised exercises specific to the involved nerves and injuries, therapy modalities to help manage symptoms, and overall lifestyle modifications. All of these efforts should help calm the nerves from the neck and brachial plexus level all the way to the hand and wrist.

The bottom line is that we need to treat thoracic outlet syndrome, carpal tunnel injuries, and repetitive strain injuries with respect. Once we acknowledge that these problems exist and are prevalent in our society, we can also accept the fact that conservative care with lifestyle and activity modification is preferable to surgery, because surgery often has less than optimal results.

2.

The Anatomy of Nerve Injury

The nerves of the arm are a wonderfully coordinated system that orchestrates activities from lifting objects to playing a piano. They allow us to experience many pleasurable things in the world, but when they are not functioning well, they can make life miserable.

The three major nerves in the arm–the median, radial, and ulnar nerves–stem from the brachial plexus. They separate into individual nerves at the shoulder level and then go into the arm, wrist, and hand (see Figure 2.1).

The median nerve provides sensation or feeling in the thumb, index, and long fingers, and in the radial half (or thumb side) of the fourth or ring finger. The median nerve also supplies motor function to those muscles, which help the hand make a fist, and to the abductor pollicis brevis muscle, which allows us to bend or oppose the thumb to the other fingers for activities such as pinching and gripping.

The ulnar nerve travels down the arm behind the elbow and into the hand, providing sensation in the pinkie and little-finger side of the ring finger. This controls dexterity and fine motor function in the hand.

The radial nerve allows us to bring our fingers out straight and the wrist back. It runs down the arm on the outside of the elbow. The radial nerve controls the extensor muscles of the forearm and also gives us sensation in the back of the hand.

Nerves can be injured anywhere from the neck to the fingertips. The brachial plexus connects the nerve roots at the neck to the upper arm and spans the gap between the neck and shoulder, and the thoracic outlet is the tunnel through which the nerves of the brachial plexus travel (see Figure 2.2). Injury to all of the nerves of the arm

17

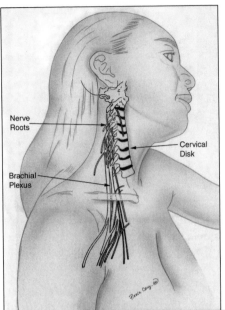

FIGURE 2.1 The cervical spine and discs are seen in their normal anatomic alignment. The nerve roots exit the spine and form the nerves of the brachial plexus. These travel through the thoracic outlet to form the major nerves of the arm.

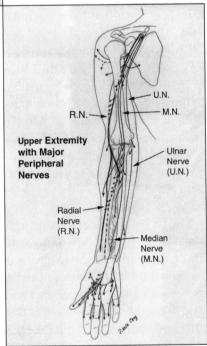

FIGURE 2.2 The nerves of the upper extremity begin as the thoracic outlet and then travel as long cables from the neck to the fingertips. The three nerves innervating the hand: the median, radial, and ulnar are seen here in their entirety. Pathology at any level can produce symptoms throughout the arm.

can occur at the thoracic outlet; alternatively, local injury can involve the ulnar or radial nerve at the elbow, or the median nerve at the carpal tunnel. More than one can be involved at the same time, which can cause overlapping and confusing symptoms.

Nerves may also be compromised above the thoracic outlet at the neck by disc herniations, where direct pressure on the nerve root decreases the ability of the nerve to conduct electricity. Discs normally act as cushions between the spinal vertebrae. If a patient has a severe whiplash-type injury, or a significant crunching or crush injury to the head and neck, the disc's soft inner material, called the nucleus pulposus, may be pushed out to the side so that it presses on the nerve root at the neck.

UNDERSTANDING YOUR NERVES

By transmitting sensory, motor, and autonomic (unconscious) impulses from one part of the body to another, the nerves allow us to interpret and react to our environment. Two types of tissues make up the nervous system. Impulse conduction tissues contain cells that transmit messages from the body to the brain and vice versa. Supportive tissues include the fascia, a form of normal scar tissue that aids in protecting the nervous system from external forces, and the blood vessels, which supply the nutrition necessary for the impulse-conducting tissues to survive.

By sliding between layers of muscle or fascia tissues, the nerves take up the slack during joint movement, which keeps them free of tension. A nerve normally enjoys considerable mobility in its bed, being only loosely attached to surrounding structures by flimsy connective tissue. This mobility minimizes the risk of a nerve sustaining a stretch injury or other type of injury. The risk of injury therefore increases when a nerve becomes firmly attached by adhesions (scar tissue) to its bed or to neighboring structures.

To function efficiently, each nerve fiber must transmit impulses at a certain speed and frequency. Since the diameter of a nerve fiber and the degree of myelination (the thickness of the sheath that surrounds the nerve) are factors influencing nerve conduction, any variance from normal could result in numbness, tingling, or pain. One type of injury that affects nerve conduction is a pinched nerve in the neck either from direct pressure or scarring about the nerve roots or thoracic outlet nerves.

A nerve's mobility and its relationship to the surrounding anatomy are crucial. A freely moving nerve may cease to function normally when it is stretched or when the surrounding structures are injured and inflamed. Scarring can impair the nerve's mobility and expose it to further damage from traction, or to injury from repeated friction.

A common example of minor nerve injury is bumping the "funny bone," or ulnar nerve, where it crosses the elbow passing into the forearm. When you bang this area you feel pain and tingling.

Nerves are also vulnerable to compression injury where they pass through a confined and crowded area bounded by unyielding walls. This can occur with the median nerve at the carpal tunnel in the wrist. Swelling and inflammation inside this closed tunnel may result in nerve symptoms well before scarring becomes an issue.

Identifying a nerve problem early on and addressing the cause can help to avoid scarring. Simply modifying the activity or environment that is causing the swelling is often enough to solve the problem.

NONSURGICAL TREATMENT OPTIONS

Most researchers who study repetitive strain, carpal tunnel and, thoracic outlet injuries in depth agree that treatment needs to begin conservatively, except in cases of severe atrophy or sensory loss. Conservative nonsurgical treatment involves gentle stretching of the involved muscles and the scar tissue surrounding the nerves. Before the onset of irritation or trauma, each patient already has his or her own individual state of muscle tension, nerve and tissue length, posture, and musculoskeletal structure. Individual predisposition, compounded by the pain of acute trauma, often results in rapid progression of contractile muscle shortening (spasm), inflammation, and the development of repetitive strain injury, carpal tunnel injury, or thoracic outlet problems.

At the Upper Extremity Institute, we have found a success rate of avoiding surgery in approximately 50 percent of patients using myriad nonsurgical treatment options. The long-term benefit is often greatest when patient education is a vital part of the program. Intelligent lifestyle choices can markedly decrease the chances for recurrence of the problem. Thorough patient education also helps those who end up needing surgery to understand that they might not get complete relief. They understand the limitations of surgery and develop realistic expectations, and they understand that continued lifestyle modification will help increase the effectiveness of their surgery.

With a modified work environment and early treatment, many nerve problems will calm down enough for the damage to be reversible. It is only when inflammation and swelling about the nerves reaches the point of significant scarring and compression that problems become permanent and require surgical intervention. This is the point when the nerves are no longer free to slide or move normally in the tissue.

Conservative treatment can include physical or occupational therapy, heat treatments, high-voltage galvanic stimulation, transcutaneous electrical nerve stimulation (TENS), acupuncture, reflexology, biofeedback, massage, shiatsu, tai chi, yoga, lifestyle and behavior modification, osteopathic and chiropractic manipulation, or other alternative therapy techniques. These therapies can be effective either with or without surgical intervention. Often changes in behavior and environment in addition to a simple wrist splint used at night are all that are required.

It is imperative that a therapy program be tailored to your individual needs as a patient and that both you and your doctor understand the nature of the symptoms. It is also essential that you understand the nature of your problem.

If your primary goal is to get relief from your symptoms, you might need to modify your work activities or, in extreme cases, consider an alternative career.

Prevention is the best "treatment" for repetitive strain injury, carpal tunnel injuries, and thoracic outlet syndrome. Once symptoms occur, don't put off seeing your doctor for diagnosis and appropriate treatment. By taking action early, you can help prevent and minimize scarring and damage while reducing the risk of permanent injury.

3.

Treatment Modalities
and How to Use Them

A variety of treatment techniques work to calm the symptoms of nerve pain and inflammation, each with its own purpose and goal. Some are quite simple, while others require advanced education and training to administer.

Heat and cold applications are often used to calm symptoms. Treatment alternatives using heat include hot packs, hot towels, warm water soaks, warm whirlpool, paraffin, fluidotherapy, ultrasound, and high-voltage galvanic stimulation. What all of these have in common is the ability to deliver heat to various depths of tissue penetration. Some therapies can reach deep tissues up to an inch and a half or so below the skin. The heat causes the blood vessels to dilate, so that they absorb and remove excess fluid in the area. This helps decrease pressure on the soft tissue structures, thus decompressing the nerves.

Cold applications work in the opposite way: A decrease in circulation from vasoconstriction reduces the amount of fluid leakage. This in turn decreases the amount of edema (swelling) or fluid secretion, which lessens the amount of fluid in the area of injury.

HEAT TREATMENTS

Heat treatment decreases stiffness by increasing tissue elasticity. It decreases pain by inhibiting the transmission of pain signals, and it decreases spasm by decreasing nerve firing. Heat treatment also increases circulation caused by dilating the blood vessels.

The best time to apply a heat treatment is before exercise. Apply it for approximately fifteen to twenty minutes, and follow with warm-ups and stretches. Anyone with circulatory problems, such as peripheral vascular disease, or with peripheral neuropathies (reduced sensation) such as that accompanying diabetes mellitus, should use extreme caution when applying heat. Those with poor circulation may have impaired ability to adjust body temperature in the arms and legs and may burn without feeling it. This is also true for others with impaired sensation to the body or the limbs, such as stroke patients. Also, patients with active clotting or bleeding problems, such as deep vein thrombosis, phlebitis, or recent bruising, should not use heat therapies.

Using heat application requires caution and common sense. Immersing a large part of the body in heat (such as a whirlpool/Jacuzzi bath) results in increased cardiac output, pulse, respiratory rate, and changes in blood pressure. Cardiac patients and others with altered ability to tolerate changes in stress on the heart should check with their doctor or therapist before initiating heat treatment.

Heat should always feel comfortable. There should be six to eight layers of toweling between hot packs and the skin. Check your skin condition and sensation before, during, and after treatment. Because the weight of a hot pack can aggravate symptoms, adjust your position so that the hot pack feels comfortable. Often a lying position works best, but if you lie on top of the hot pack, use extra layers of toweling to prevent burns.

〵   〵   〵

The following types of heat therapies can be used at home. Be sure to follow the manufacturer's guidelines regarding the use and appropriateness of any particular treatment.

HOT PACKS

A pack, often canvas, filled with gel or sand is heated by immersing it in water or in a microwave oven. Many variations are available, filled with various substances and imparting different levels of heat for varying periods of time. Some even provide aromatherapy as well.

HOT TOWELS

These are moistened towels designed to be heated in a microwave oven. Patients with potential circulatory or skin complications should use extra layers of dry toweling to prevent burns. Figures 3.1 and 3.2 show examples of appropriately applied hot packs.

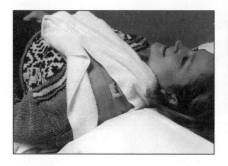 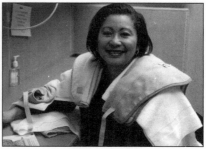

FIGURE 3.1   A patient with a hot pack appropriately applied.

FIGURE 3.2   Another view of appropriately applied hot packs.

WARM WATER SOAKS OR WARM WHIRLPOOL

With the water temperature typically at about 100 degrees F., a soak in a regular or whirlpool bath can be used in conjunction with active exercise in the water to decrease pain and stiffness (see Figure 3.3). When using a whirlpool, try to adjust the agitation according to your individual sensitivity. When using either a whirlpool or a basin for a warm water soak, avoid putting pressure on potential pressure points, such as the wrist or elbow, by putting a pad or towel on the edge or simply being careful not to rest the arm on the edge while bathing the affected area. This helps to maximize comfort and prevent compression on nerves and blood vessels.

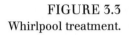

FIGURE 3.3
Whirlpool treatment.

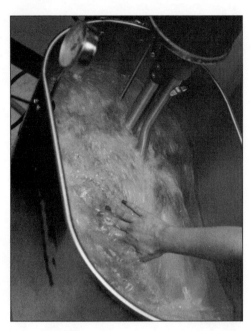

PARAFFIN

This is a liquid wax with mineral oil, mixed in a 6:1 ratio. If paraffin proves to be effective for you, you might want to obtain your own unit for home use from a local surgical supply store. Some beauty and health salons even have these available, but check with your therapist or doctor before trying it.

For applying heat to the hand, paraffin is often more effective than a hot pack. The wax can form to the small joints in your fingers and hands and surround them with comforting warmth. Before dipping your hand in the paraffin, remove all jewelry or secure it in place with gauze. Place your hand in the paraffin for one to two seconds, and do this six to twelve times to form layers. To prevent burns, be careful not to touch the sides or the bottom of the container. Check the skin before and after use. After all of the layers of paraffin are on, wrap the wrist and hand in a plastic bag, plastic wrap, or waxed paper secured with loose tape or a rubber band, then wrap all of this in a towel. For increased heat, you can add a hot pack to the paraffin wrap after wrapping it in plastic. The heating effect usually lasts twenty to thirty minutes, after which you easily peel away the wax and discard it. Figures 3.4–3.6 show a typical paraffin application to the hand.

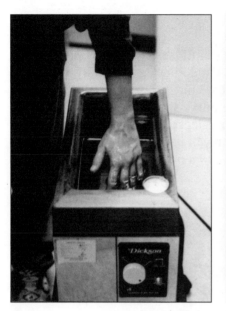

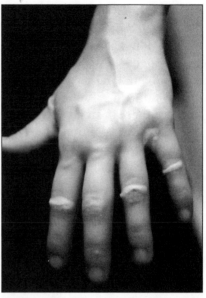

FIGURE 3.4 Paraffin treatment, step one: Dip the hand into the hot paraffin.

FIGURE 3.5 Paraffin treatment, step two: Remove the hand. This closeup shows coverage with wax.

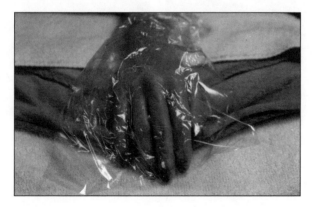

FIGURE 3.6 Paraffin treatment, optional step three: Plastic wrap with additional heat.

FLUIDOTHERAPY

Circulation of heated silicon or cellulose particles creates a dry whirlpool effect with this therapy. Fluidotherapy is usually applied in a therapy unit, using a relatively large machine that is admittedly not ideally suited for home use (see Figures 3.7 and 3.8). You place your arm or other affected area through a sleeve, where it rests in the dried particles. The area under treatment can be held stationary or used in combination with gentle exercise to decrease stiffness or pain. It can also be used for desensitization.

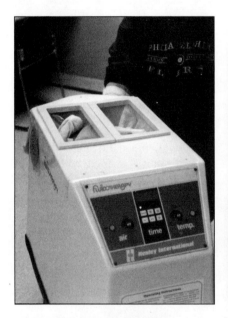

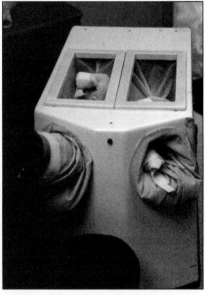

FIGURE 3.7   The fluidotherapy machine.

FIGURE 3.8   Fluidotherapy treatment. The patient inserts his or her arm(s) into the padded collar(s).

The following deep-heating therapies generally need to be applied in a clinical setting, by a doctor or therapist with special training.

ULTRASOUND

An ultrasound device's applicator contains a crystal that converts electrical energy into acoustical energy. The power generated causes the crystal inside the applicator to vibrate and produce sound waves, which penetrate to approximately one inch below the skin. The thermal effect of therapeutic ultrasound helps to decrease pain, stiffness, and muscle spasms. It also helps increase circulation. When used at relatively low intensities and on a pulsed mode, ultrasound also helps decrease swelling through a mechanical effect that causes streaming of fluid molecules.

Prior to performing ultrasound, the clinician applies a gel to the affected area, because ultrasound waves travel through gel better than through air (see Figures 3.9 and 3.10). The clinician then applies the ultrasound applicator to the skin and moves it continuously to prevent burning. This lasts for anywhere from three to ten minutes. If the affected area is not relatively flat, ultrasound can be used in water to make it easier to keep the ultrasound head in contact with skin

Sometimes you can detect a mild heating sensation, but usually you don't feel the heating effect while ultrasound is being applied. If you

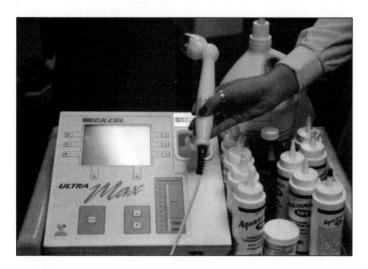

FIGURE 3.9   Ultrasound unit. The bottles shown at right contain gels and optional medication.

begin to feel an uncomfortable heating sensation, you should tell the therapist so that he or she can change the intensity and mode.

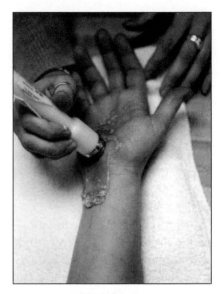

FIGURE 3.10   Application of ultrasound to the carpal tunnel.

When ultrasound is used in conjunction with topical medications, the deep heating effect of the ultrasound helps drive medication into the affected tissues to help relieve symptoms. The delivery of medication via ultrasound is called phonophoresis. It involves applying a cream–often a cortisone preparation–directly to the skin before applying the ultrasound gel. Cortisone has an anti-inflammatory effect that helps to relieve pain and swelling. Lidocaine, an anesthetic, may also be used for pain relief.

Some patients have allergic sensitivities to the medication or to the ultrasound current, so you and your therapist should watch for rashes, color changes, or swelling that can occur during or after treatment.

ELECTRICAL MODALITIES

TENS and "Hi-Volt" units are often helpful for decreasing pain. These are used in a clinical setting, but some patients learn how to set them up at home.

Various theories that explain why electrical stimulation may calm pain are not necessarily mutually exclusive and may have combined influences on pain perception:

First, the body is capable of releasing its own pain-relieving substances, called endorphins, enkephalins, and serotonin. Electrical modalities might directly stimulate this release.

Second, the "gate control" theory of pain control proposes that using sensory stimulation inhibits the propagation of messages along pain-conducting fibers. In other words, sensory stimulation of the electrical stimulation unit "blocks" your body's perception of the pain by blocking transmission of the pain signal to the brain.

A third explanation, which could apply to acupuncture as well, involves overstimulation. When the nerve fibers are forced to fire continuously, it exhausts the amount of neurotransmitter available to send impulses across the synapses—the connecting points between nerve cells. Continuous stimulation of the nerves to fire the impulses depletes the transmitter substance and weakens the signal, so that pain decreases as the signal weakens.

HIGH-VOLTAGE STIMULATION

High-voltage galvanic stimulation/direct current stimulation is a common electrical modality used to decrease pain, inflammation, or spasm. It can also be used for strengthening muscles, stimulating nerves to maintain muscle function while nerves regenerate, healing wounds, and increasing mobility.

The therapist first prepares the skin with alcohol or a hot pack to decrease any resistance (from sweat or surface dirt), then places active treatment electrodes on the skin in areas where symptoms are present. The therapist next places a larger dispersive electrode on an area with a large skin surface, such as the low back, thigh, calf, upper arm, or forearm. The dispersive electrode does not actively treat the patient but has a grounding effect to complete the circuit. All electrodes are hooked into the E-stim (electrical stimulation) unit by leads or wires.

When the E-stim unit is turned on, the patient should experience a comfortable tingling sensation. There should be no muscular response or contraction. The E-stim should feel comfortable, and its intensity should feel strong but tolerable.

E-stim works primarily by inhibiting the transmission of pain signals to the brain. It also activates muscle pumping actions that push fluid out of the area to decrease swelling, and it can decrease spasm by fatiguing the muscles.

E-stim is not used over healing fractures, areas with tendency to bleed or clot, tumors, phlebitis, superficial metal implants, pacemakers, or on patients with heart disease. E-stim is also inappropriate for use on the head, face, abdomen, chest, front of the neck, vital organs, and spinal cord. It is not advised for patients with epilepsy, stroke, or recent scars or sutures, nor is it recommended for patients with decreased sensation, severe swelling, cuts, rashes, bruises, or sensitivity to electrical current.

The patient and therapist check the skin before, during, and after treatment to observe possible discoloration or swelling. They should also examine the E-stim unit for any broken or frayed wires before and after treatment and avoid using any damaged equipment.

IONTOPHORESIS

Iontophoresis is the application of a continuous direct current that assists in transferring medication through the skin to decrease pain or inflammation. It is based on the concept of differential ion shifts caused by electrical current shifting. Iontophoresis units work on batteries, and their very low voltage helps ensure safety.

One commonly used medication is the cortisone preparation Dexamethasone, an anti-inflammatory that helps reduce pain and swelling. Another is Lidocaine, an anesthetic that helps to reduce pain.

The procedure for iontophoresis is similar to that used for E-stim, except that medication is applied to the electrodes before they are placed on the skin. Contraindications are similar to those for E-stim, and some patients are allergic or sensitive to certain medications. It should not be used near open wounds.

TRANSCUTANEOUS ELECTRICAL NERVE STIMULATION (TENS)

TENS is similar in effect to the high-voltage pulse current/electrical stimulation, but it works by overstimulating the nerves and depleting the amount of neurotransmitter available at the nerve synapses. This causes a decrease in the amount and intensity of pain signals sent to the brain and stimulates the body to produce its own natural painkillers (endorphins and enkephalins).

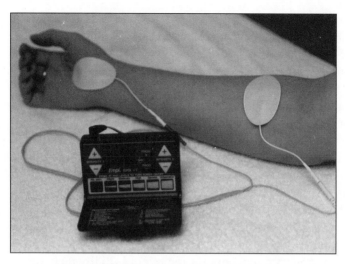

FIGURE 3.11 A TENS unit is applied.

TENS does not help to reduce inflammation, but it may have a similar effect by reducing muscle spasm. Rather than using a dispersive pad, the therapist or patient places active treatment electrodes directly onto the areas where symptoms occur (see Figures 3.11 and 3.12).

Initially, the therapist or doctor sets the rate of stimulation of TENS in the clinic. If TENS proves to be effective for you, discuss the possibility of acquiring a unit for home use. Once you are comfortable with its use at home, you can adjust the rate according to your needs.

Contraindications and precautions are the same as those for electrical stimulation.

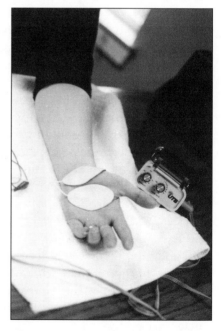

FIGURE 3.12 A high-voltage unit is applied.

COLD APPLICATIONS

Treatments involving cold application include cold packs and ice packs, iced towels, contrast baths, cold water soaks, cold whirlpool, and ice massage. Cold is generally used after exercise to decrease pain or swelling, but it can be used prior to exercise if there is significant swelling or pain, or if it is used simply for pain control.

The age-old advice about when to use ice or heat with an acute injury is relatively simple: Use ice for the first twenty-four hours and then use either ice or heat, whichever feels better.

Cold treatment decreases pain by inhibiting the transmission of pain signals. It also helps to decrease swelling by constricting the blood vessels, and it helps decrease muscle spasm.

When using cold treatment, the patient initially feels the sensation of cold, followed by a burning sensation. Next comes an aching sensation, and finally a numbing of the area. Typically, all of these steps occur within ten to fifteen minutes.

Cold therapy is not recommended for anyone with impaired sensation or circulation problems, including patients with stroke, peripheral vascular disease, diabetes mellitus, or sensitivity to cold from Raynaud's disease or scleroderma. Cold can also cause hives or flushing of the skin, and it can result in decreased heart rate, increased cardiac output, drop in blood pressure, or difficulty breathing.

Precautions include joint stiffness and decreased circulation, so the patient and therapist should be cautious about initiating cold treatment before exercise. Also, prolonged application of cold over superficial nerves—at the elbow, for example—can cause numbness, tingling, and discomfort. Precautions involving the weight of a cold pack are similar to those for heat therapy. You or your doctor should inspect your skin before, during, and after treatment and remove all jewelry.

In addition, be aware of a hunting reaction, which is a protective response of the body in which blood vessels alternately dilate and constrict after prolonged exposure to cold. This may be painful. If you experience this, stop using the cold modality until your therapist or doctor can evaluate it.

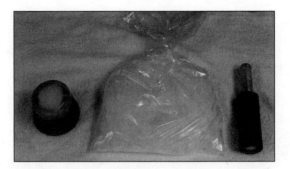

FIGURE 3.13   Three types of ice application.
From left, the ice cup, crushed ice in a bag, and
the ice pen.

COLD PACKS AND ICE PACKS

One of the simplest cold treatments is a vinyl or plastic cold pack
filled with gel. You cover it with a towel or pillowcase to protect the
skin and apply it for ten to fifteen minutes. Never apply a cold pack
directly to the skin. Alternatively, you can make an ice pack. Simply
place crushed or cubed ice in a plastic bag, wrap it in cloth, and apply
it for ten to fifteen minutes. Figure 3.13 shows an ice pack and two
other types of ice application.

ICED TOWELS

Another method of applying cold is with iced towels. Dip terrycloth
towels in slushy water with crushed or cubed ice, wring out the excess water, then apply the towel to the skin for ten to fifteen minutes.

COLD WATER SOAKS AND WHIRLPOOLS

A cold water bath or whirlpool at approximately 60 degrees F. helps
reduce pain and inflammation if you combine it with an in-water exercise program. Slowly move your fingers and the area where symp-

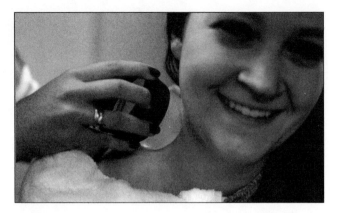

FIGURE 3.14 Ice massage can be very effective in calming muscle spasm. Shown is the ice cup application.

toms are occurring for ten to fifteen minutes. The agitation action of a whirlpool can help cleanse a wound and desensitize the area.

Pressure points where the elbow and wrist meet the edges of the whirlpool should be padded with a towel to decrease risk of compression of vessels and nerves.

CONTRAST BATHS

A contrast bath, involving alternate immersion in warm and cold water, is very effective for reducing swelling, especially if it is acute. Treatment begins with immersion of the affected area in warm water (approximately 100 degrees F.) for two minutes. This is followed by one minute in cold water (about 50 degrees F.), then another two minutes in warm water, one minute in cold water, and so on, for a total of twenty minutes, ending with the warm water immersion.

Using this in conjunction with nerve sliding or tendon gliding exercises can further decrease pain and inflammation.

ICE MASSAGE

Ice massage is often more effective than a cold pack for treating small areas, such as the base of the thumb, or over the long thoracic nerve

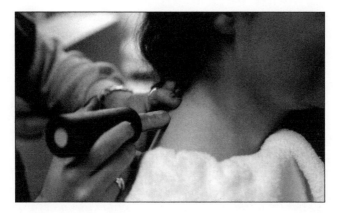

FIGURE 3.15   The ice pen can be used to treat smaller areas or "trigger points."

in the upper back. It gives a more intense, directed local effect than you get from a cold pack.

To use ice massage at home, fill a Styrofoam or paper cup with water and place a popsicle stick or tongue depressor inside. Freeze, then peel away the cup and rub the ice directly over the painful or swollen area with circular, overlapping strokes for five to ten minutes. (If you don't use a stick or tongue depressor, peel away only the bottom half of the cup to expose the ice. Continue rubbing until the area is numb or the ice begins to melt. On hot days you may need to refreeze, or use a second application, if the ice melts too quickly. Figures 3.14 and 3.15 show an ice cup application as well as office treatment using an ice pen.

MEDICATIONS

Although they are not the first line of treatment choice, medication therapy may be a worthwhile addition to your home program. I recommend using them relatively sparingly, but they are often a useful adjunct, especially on days when symptoms flare up severely.

Medication should be an adjunct to a well-oriented treatment program, not a substitute for good care: Do not use it so that you can allow continued abuse of your body. Medication is, however, often helpful in treating many of the symptoms of nerve disease and injury. Discuss appropriate types and doses with your doctor or pharmacist.

Nonsteroidal anti-inflammatory medications such as Motrin, Advil, Nuprin, and Naproxen are often helpful for decreasing swelling and pain. They work by inhibiting the production of prostaglandins. Aspirin is also a very good, time-tested anti-inflammatory agent for many individuals. It works somewhat differently than the nonsteroidals. New prescription nonsteroidal anti-inflammatory medications include Celebrex and Vioxx, which have the advantage of being absorbed in the intestine rather than the stomach and are reported to have fewer gastric upset effects. Each of the anti-inflammatory medications is slightly different, so if one does not work for you, it may be worthwhile to try another.

Tylenol, or acetaminophen, is a very good pain reliever that can have fewer side effects than the anti-inflammatory medications. It does not relieve inflammation.

Narcotic medications, such as Darvocet, Percocet, Percodan, and extended release oxycontin are often helpful if used judiciously for breaking the pain spasm cycle to initiate long-term reduction of symptoms. They are addictive and should only be used under a doctor's supervision and for appropriate periods of time.

Muscle relaxers, such as Flexeril, Valium, Xanax, or a glass of beer or table wine, are also very good adjuncts to the treatment of muscle spasm and nerve pain. They help to break the spasm of muscles around the nerves, thereby reducing local inflammation and disruption of axonal flow associated with nerve pain. They are especially helpful at night for decreasing pain and improving sleep, but they should be used judiciously.

Antidepressant medications such as Elavil, Buspar, and Prozac have been proven effective in decreasing the amount of neurotransmitter secreted by nerves, thus helping to decrease nerve pain. They often have the side effect of helping to restore regular sleep patterns, and they can be beneficial in cases of low-lying appropriate reactive depression. It is important to remember that these medications have withdrawal effects and should be discontinued slowly, under the guidance of your physician, with both of you determining the appropriate timing.

4.

A Nerve Sliding Program

The best way to prevent scar tissue from constricting motion and function is to keep the structures moving. If a car is left in a garage for a long period of time and then taken out on the road, it is likely to run poorly and need work to free frozen parts and clogged hoses. If, on the other hand, it is first prepared for storage, and run intermittently while being stored, such problems can be avoided.

Physicians have learned from orthopedic experience with knee and joint replacements that the sooner a patient begins motion after the surgery, the better the result and the fewer the complications.

For nerve injuries as well, the key to the success of any therapy program is motion–soon after the injury or surgery, to help prevent of the formation of constricting scar tissue. This is why understanding and incorporating a nerve sliding program is vital to the treatment of nerve injury at all levels.

Our treatment approach at the Upper Extremity Institute incorporates five basic principles and goals: (1) decrease the pain; (2) relax the muscles; (3) learn and incorporate a stretching and nerve sliding protocol; (4) correct the posture; and (5) educate the patient in the pathology and in the healing process.

Important elements of treatment therefore include:

- A progressive stretching and exercise program specific to the muscles of the neck and upper extremities
- Postural awareness and correction to protect the nerves and keep them in positions for optimal healing and function
- Lifestyle and activity modifications to take some stress off the affected nerves

- Adjustment of workplace ergonomics to help prevent further nerve trauma

NERVE SLIDING

The concept of nerve sliding or gliding is often confusing to patients. The nerves become bound, or stuck, when encased in the scar tissue that forms in the soft tissues surrounding them. Nerve scarring is believed to result when the nerve is not able to slide through the surrounding tissues, or when the tissues themselves are unable to slide over or across the nerve. This makes normal movement of the neck and arm painful and restricted.

Because the nerves run through muscular and soft tissue beds, they are not rigidly held in the tissues. Rather, they slide just as tendons slide. Pathology and dysfunction result when they are not allowed to slide freely. In the past we imagined the nerves sliding between the tissues, but we now realize that what is really happening is a differential sliding between the nerves and the surrounding tissues.

Nerve sliding is a more accurate term for what has in the past been called nerve gliding. Similar exercises have been described by Dr. James Hunter et al. in *Rehabilitation of the Hand: Surgery and Therapy*, fourth edition (1995). Our program expands on these basic tenants and incorporates the understanding that it is not just the nerve sliding but rather a differential slide between the nerve and its surrounding tissues.

The nerves run primarily in beds between muscle layers. When the arm is brought out and away from the body, the nerves themselves need to accommodate the change in the length or distance from the body. We now understand that rather than gliding through the tissues, the nerves stay at their fixed length as the tissues around them slide over the nerves. Trying to stretch the nerves can result in pain, discomfort, and even injury.

When you perform nerve sliding exercises, you are allowing the soft tissues surrounding the nerves to move more easily over the surface of the nerves. You can avoid permanent scarring by allowing the early "sticky tissue" or inflammation to calm down and not congeal about the nerves. If the nerves do not become permanently scarred, long-term fixed nerve problems will not occur.

This concept applies whether you subscribe to the theory that nerve problems are caused strictly by compression or believe that they are a result of scarring and inability of nerves to slide through the tissues. Sliding helps reduce inflammation. If scarring or inflammation is present, gentle stretching will help reduce inflammation and the possibility of permanent scarring.

Our unique approach to moving the nerves by gently sliding them through the surrounding tissues helps to maintain blood supply to the nerves and improve their mobility. This sliding also stretches out any early-forming scar tissue caused by inflammation, so that the scar tissue will not permanently constrict the nerves.

Following is the correct technique for completing a "slide" of each of the major nerves in the arm, as well as a general "slide" for the brachial plexus nerves. None of these movements should cause pain or numbness. You should begin each exercise slowly and stop if you experience any numbness, tingling, or pain. Mild discomfort that resolves upon completion of the exercise is appropriate in patients with significant nerve injury, but continued pain or symptoms mean that you are doing too much. If you experience a slight pull, discomfort, or tingling, back off slightly.

BRACHIAL PLEXUS SLIDING

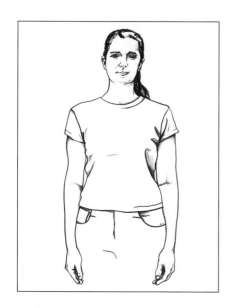

The goal here is to move the nerves and their extensions down the entire length of the arm. This sequence should be performed slowly. This series of movements will gradually slide the nerves in the arm and hand through their surrounding soft tissue.

Begin with the head facing forward, ears aligned over shoulders, and spine in good posture as shown at left.

Step one. Bend the elbow comfortably in front of your body, with your wrist also slightly bent in a flexed or downward position and your head slightly tilted toward the shoulder of the arm that is in front of you.

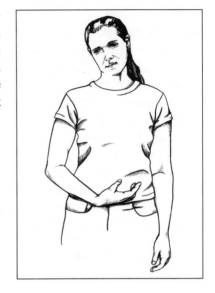

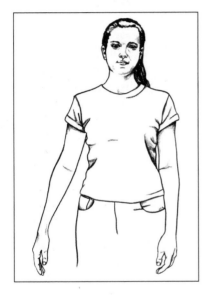

Step two. Slowly straighten your arm; bring your lower arm further out away from you (to the side), downward and in front of your body. Bring your head straight up to neutral.

Step three. Begin to straighten your wrist to neutral (up from bent down), with your elbow nearly straight and the arm out away from your body. Reminder: only go to the point of gentle stretch.

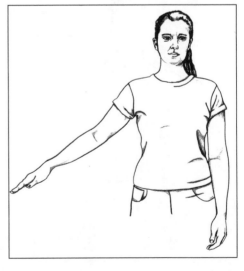

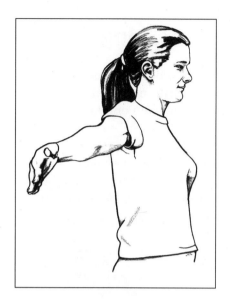

Step four. Move your wrist back to a slight extension. Bring your arm gradually away from your body and back, until it is slightly below shoulder height and slightly behind your body (*top*). At this point, if you have no discomfort or symptoms, tilt your head slowly toward the affected side and slightly extend your wrist (*middle*). Then tilt your head away from the affected arm, simultaneously flexing your wrist (*bottom*). Next, slowly, reverse this motion one more time. Reminder: In the final stage, do not hold your arm in the air for more than thirty seconds

This is the maximum stretch recommended for the plexus. You should feel a gentle stretch, with no symptoms of pain, tingling, or numbness.

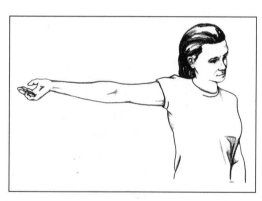

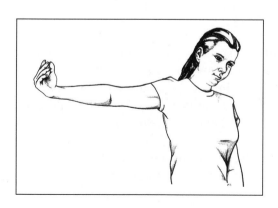

RADIAL NERVE SLIDING

This slide is best performed while standing, but you can perform it while seated if your chair allows for arm movement. Try to reach a point of stretch with some tension but no pain or other symptoms.

Step one.   Stand in good posture and relax. Press the involved shoulder gently downward, as if you are reaching for a small object on the floor (*below left*). Straighten the elbow with your hand by your side (*below right*). You should not feel a stretch or tension response. If you do, back off until you reach your comfort zone.

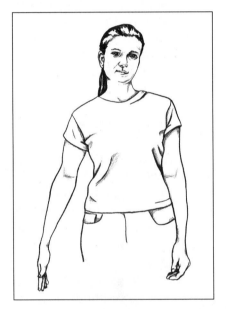
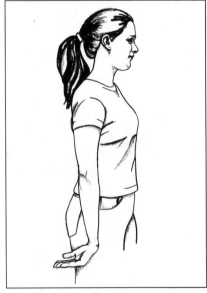

Step two.   With your shoulder depressed, bend your wrist down into slight flexion, and rotate your arm inward (with your thumb toward your body). This position is sometimes referred to as the "waiter's tip" posture, with the hand out behind the body as if secretly waiting to have someone place money in the hand (*opposite, top*).

Step three.   While maintaining the above position, slide the radial nerve further by tilting your head toward the depressed shoulder.

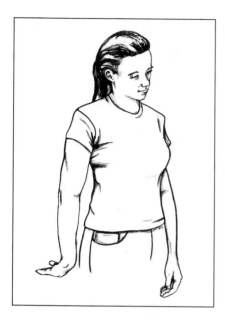

Then tilt your head away from the involved arm while simultaneously extending your wrist (*below left*). Slowly reverse this motion at the neck and wrist one more time.

Step four. Bend the wrist further back and extend your arm behind your body slightly (*below right*). Remember that more is not necessarily better. This should be a gentle slide of the radial nerve through the surrounding soft tissues.

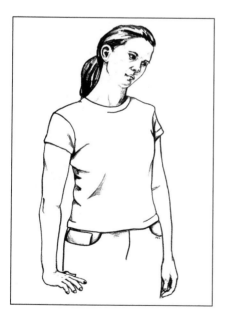

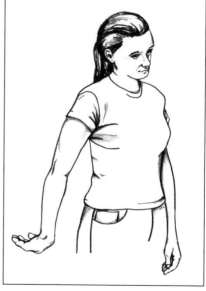

As with all of these exercises, if you feel any new symptoms tell your doctor or therapist at your next visit.

ULNAR NERVE SLIDING

The same principles for sliding apply to the ulnar nerve. The elbow is a typical area of involvement for this "funny bone" nerve, which travels behind the bone on the inside of the elbow. If there is inadequate ability for the nerve to make the trip behind the bone when the elbow is bent or flexed, it may be stretched or even pop out of the groove and produce symptoms.

SERIES 1: SLIDING THE ULNAR NERVE DISTALLY, OR THROUGH THE LOWER ARM AND HAND

Step one. Begin with the ulnar nerve in a slackened position. Keep your arm straight in front of you, below the height of your shoulder, and flex your wrist up toward the ceiling, with the palm facing you.

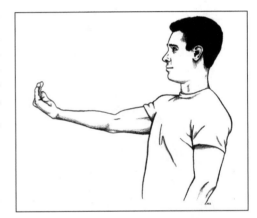

Step two. Bend your wrist back and downward toward the floor (into extension), and straighten your fingers. Begin to bend your elbow slightly.

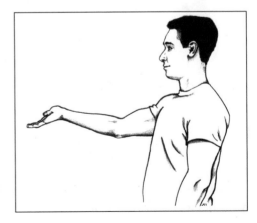

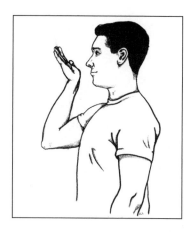

Step three. Maintain this position of your wrist and hand while slowly bending your elbow, bringing the heel (palm) of your hand in toward your chin. This series slides the ulnar nerve along the lower part of your arm.

SERIES 2: SLIDING THE ULNAR NERVE PROXIMALLY– ABOVE THE LEVEL OF THE ELBOW

Depending on where your restrictions lie, this set of exercises may produce more tension in your arm than do the radial nerve sliding exercises. If you find that both slides are appropriate for you, you may benefit from performing one right after the other.

Step one. Extend your arm straight out to the side of your body, slightly below shoulder height, with your palm facing downward. Your elbow and wrist should be straight, and your fingers should be curled slightly.

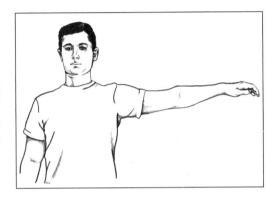

Step two. Bend your wrist slightly while rolling your arm over to turn your palm upward. This adds tension to the nerve. You should feel stretch, not pain.

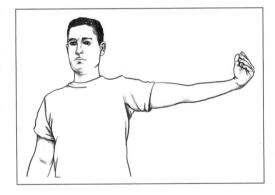

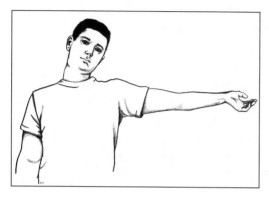

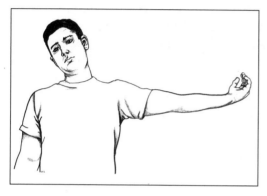

Step three. While maintaining the above position, bend your neck toward the side of your outstretched arm at the same time you extend your wrist (*top*). This produces a gentle pull on the upper portion of the nerve at the lower brachial plexus as it travels through the axilla (armpit). Next bend your neck away from the arm and simultaneously flex your wrist (*bottom*).

Slowly reverse this motion at the neck and wrist one more time.

SERIES 3: MEDIAN NERVE SLIDING

The median nerve begins at the neck at the C-5/6 nerve root and travels through the brachial plexus. It terminates at the carpal tunnel at the wrist, where it is at high risk for injury. These slides address the nerve at its most distal level, the carpal tunnel. It also addresses the underlying problem in many early carpal tunnel nerve injuries: tendinitis, or swelling of the lining around the flexor tendons. These exercises help to decrease the inflammation and slide the tendons as well as the nerve, a double plus for healing.

You can perform this slide while sitting or lying down. Begin with your upper body in good posture with your arm at your side and elbow bent at a 90-degree angle.

Step one. With your wrist straight (neutral), hold your fingers and thumb in a relaxed closed fist with your fingernails facing you (*left*),

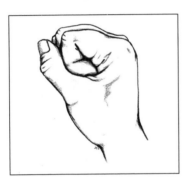
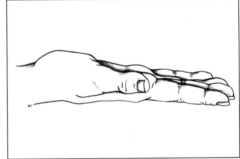

then slowly, with mild tension, straighten your fingers and thumb (*right*).

Step two. Extend your wrist back, keeping your fingers straight, and turn your forearm so that your palm is facing upward, toward the sky.

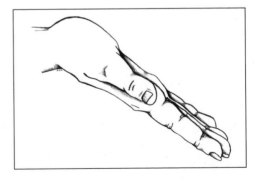

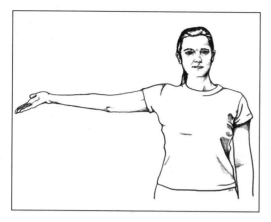

Step three. While maintaining the above position, give a gentle extra stretch to the fingers to bring them out completely straight to "flatten out" your hand (*opposite, bottom*).

Step four. To stretch the median nerve in the upper arm, bring the arm out to the side. Slowly extend or straighten the elbow and bring the arm up to shoulder height (*left*). You should feel a gentle stretch in the forearm. Do not overdo this. If you are comfortable with this after a few sessions, you may add a lateral tilt of the head away from the outstretched arm to complete the stretch at the brachial plexus level.

❧   ❧   ❧

Begin with five to ten repetitions of each exercise, pausing between repetitions. Initially, do the series three times a day, then gradually add more sessions throughout the day or increase the length of each session, without overdoing it. The key to improvement is slow, steady movement, with respect for the delicate and intricate structure of the nerves.

5.

Soft Tissue Stretching

Many cases of repetitive strain injury, carpal tunnel problems, and thoracic outlet syndrome will resolve with appropriate stretching and sliding exercises. The type and angle of stretch and the degree of pull are critical, however.

Most patients require several sessions of exacting instruction. Be cautious when stretching the upper extremity muscles, because the process literally pulls the already tight, shortened, or contracted muscles and soft tissue structures against the neurovascular bundle or the brachial plexus. In addition, the nerves themselves are sensitive and can be a direct source of pain when stretched. This is why, in most cases, it is better to stretch yourself rather than have someone else pull or stretch your tissues.

Effective therapeutic stretching needs to be gradual and progressive. Each stretch session need last only a few minutes, so that doing stretches ten times daily may amount to a total of only thirty minutes a day. Although you may initially feel some "stretch discomfort," symptoms should subside within seconds or minutes following the stretch. There should be no residual pain after stretching.

Remember to keep breathing while performing all exercises. Holding your breath while concentrating on a movement can increase your blood pressure and encourage tension in the muscles. It also decreases the oxygen flow to your bloodstream, causing a real decrease in the available nutrition needed for the muscles and nerves to respond appropriately to the challenge of stretching and healing.

Following are some basic exercises that you can begin at home. They are specific to the muscles of the neck and arm, which are often tight or tense. The upper trapezius muscle works to draw the scapula or shoulder blade upward. This is the muscle that allows us to shrug our shoulders. It is a common site of spasm and tightness. The scalene muscles, located between the neck and shoulder, surround and support the brachial plexus, so it is imperative for these muscles to be stretched with great caution. Tightness of the scalenes can contribute to thoracic outlet syndrome because of pressure from short or tense muscles.

START POSITION

To begin any type of stretch, sit in good posture with your low back supported. Try performing these stretches in front of a mirror so that you can check your posture. Face forward with your ears aligned over your shoulders. Sit in a supportive chair with arm rests positioned to support the arms while you relax the nerves in the upper extremities. The arm rests should be positioned in such a manner so that you can raise or lower your shoulders in a way that feels natural. Allow enough time to perform the exercises slowly while you are relaxed.

LATERAL NECK STRETCH

Beginning in proper start position, bring your ear toward your shoulder until you feel a comfortable pull or stretch. As you move your head toward the shoulder, do not bring your shoulder up. Look forward and hold for a slow count of ten. Remember to keep the stretch comfortable.

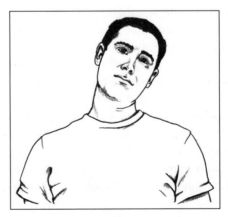

SHOULDER ROLLS

From proper start position, slowly raise your shoulders up toward your ears. Very slowly, rotate your shoulders backward, gently squeezing the shoulder blades together, then rotate your shoulders downward, to the lowest point comfortable. Continue rotating your shoulders, making the widest circle comfortable. Perform five to ten complete revolutions. This exercise provides a gentle stretch to the muscles surrounding the shoulders and neck.

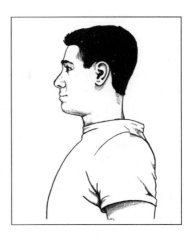

ANTERIOR NECK STRETCHES

Step one. Beginning in proper start position, slowly bring one ear towards your shoulder, away from the affected side.

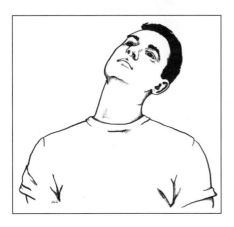

Step two. Before a stretch point is reached, slowly rotate your face up toward the ceiling so that you are looking upward in a side-type glance to the opposite side of the stretch, until a soft, gentle stretch is felt on the side and front of your neck. This should feel very comfortable. Gently hold for a slow count of ten.

If your symptoms are reproduced or exacerbated, you have gone too far. This is an excellent stretch for the anterior scalene muscle proper.

NECK ROTATION

This exercise incorporates many of the muscles that support the neck and shoulders.

Beginning in proper start position, slowly rotate your head, looking to the left or right, keeping your eyes level.

Bring your nose down toward your shoulder until you feel a gentle stretch. Hold for a slow count of ten.

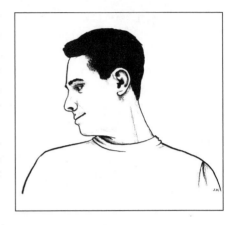

CHIN TUCKS

This exercise is one of my favorites. When performed correctly, it is a terrific stretch for the postural muscles and the cervical spine. It is especially good for those who tend to assume a "forward" head posture, as many of us do when reading or sitting for prolonged periods.

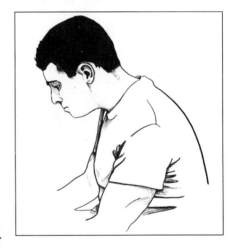

It is easy to recognize the stress this puts on our necks when we closely evaluate this posture. The chin tuck exercise stretches the posterior aspect of the lower cervical spine, which often is shortened and tight because of the tendency to stress these muscles in daily life to maintain an upright position of the head.

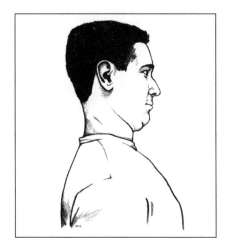

Step one. Begin in proper start position. While keeping your head level, slowly bring your chin in, producing a double chin. Your head should not tilt up or down. Feel a gentle pull in the back of the neck. Depending on your tissue restrictions and tightness, you may feel this down to the region between your shoulder blades. You are more likely to feel this down your upper back in the shoulder blade region if you have long thoracic nerve involvement off the upper trunk of your brachial plexus. This exercise helps to stretch the nerve as well as the muscles.

Step two. If this is comfortable, continue the stretch by bending the head forward and looking down slightly.

Adding self-massage to your neck helps to make this and the other neck stretches more effective. Pause briefly, then relax before repeating. Remember to keep the stretch comfortable.

6.

Posture Do's and Don'ts

When you stand up straight rather than slouching, your bones and muscles fall into their natural alignment, which helps your nerves to pass through the body unimpeded. Many of us assume poor posture out of habit. We commonly keep the head too far forward and round the shoulders, or raise them, which puts significant strain on the neck muscles and the brachial plexus nerve complex (see Figure 6.1).

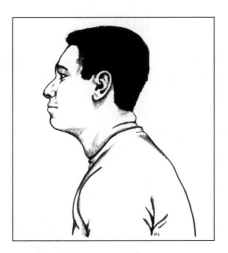

FIGURE 6.1   Forward Head Posture with Rounded Shoulders

SITTING POSTURE

Sitting correctly is the first rule of comfort. Keep your head and neck upright, with your ears directly over your shoulders (see Figure 6.2). This helps maintain proper alignment of the neck and the entire spine. Try to be continually aware of how you are sitting. Stiffness and soreness are apt to result from letting yourself slouch or reach too far forward, which causes significant strain on the structures of the brachial plexus and the nerves in the lower arm at the elbow and carpal tunnel.

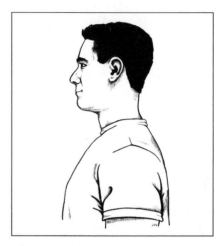

FIGURE 6.2   Correct Posture

DRIVING

While driving, hold the steering wheel low, rather than at the middle or top, in order to minimize stress on the nerves in your arms (see Figure 6.3). Hold it securely, but try to relax the arms and hands. During long trips, you may want to rest your forearm on a pillow for support.

Make sure your car seat offers good low back support to allow correct sitting posture. Keeping the low back or lumbar spine in proper posture translates up the rest of your spine to help keep

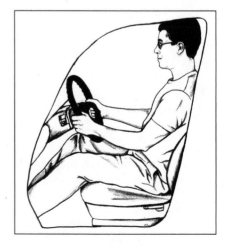

FIGURE 6.3   When Driving, Try to Relax Your Arms and Hands but Maintain Control of the Wheel

your body properly aligned. Automobiles vary tremendously with respect to seating comfort, so when shopping for a car, you should carefully evaluate how your body fits the seat. Remember also that the use of a standard shifter requires a good deal of regular reaching and use of the left leg.

Driving can lead to neck and brachial plexus pain from prolonged posturing of the neck and shoulders, as well as the constant need to turn and stretch the neck from side to side. Try to use mirrors to help minimize strain.

On extended trips, take turns with other drivers and stop frequently to rest your eyes and to do stretches and nerve slides. I generally recommend stopping every thirty to sixty minutes, depending on the severity of your symptoms. Break up long trips by stopping at rest stops, or a hotel overnight, rather than overstraining from fatigue and prolonged stress.

Whenever staying away from home, consider bringing your own pillows.

SLEEPING

The average person spends about a third of their life in bed. Appropriate sleep postures and bedding can therefore make a great difference in the healing process. Furthermore, lack of sleep and poor ability to rest significantly impact a person's ability to heal. Fatigue is the number-one complaint of my patients who have long-term nerve injury. In fact, poor sleep and lack of exercise make many people with low-level nerve injury significantly more disabled than they might otherwise be.

Certain sleeping positions can exacerbate the symptoms of repetitive strain injury, carpal tunnel problems, fibromyalgia joint pain, and thoracic outlet syndrome. If there is strain on irritated tissues during sleep, those tissues will not have an opportunity to rest and begin healing.

The position that is best for your body is often a matter of personal preference, but some general guidelines will help you find the most appropriate ones for you. As your condition improves, you may find that some postures are more effective than others for relieving your discomfort.

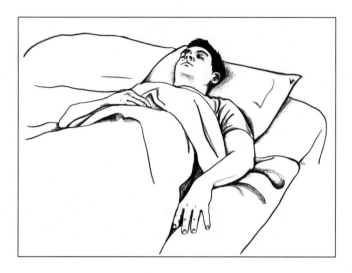

FIGURE 6.4   Proper Sleep Position Varies, but Try to
Avoid Undue Stress on Your Arms and Neck

We do things to ourselves in our sleep that we would never do
while awake. We assume awkward postures and at times perform
movements that can cause injury. Never watch television lying on a
couch with your arm under your head, or with the neck kinked, and
be sure not to fall asleep in that position too. Try to avoid sleeping on
your arm at any time, because the direct pressure of your weight can
cause nerve injury.

Sleeping on your back is probably the most orthopedically correct
posture. Even if you have no nerve injury, try not to use more than
one supporting pillow under your head. Your neck needs to remain in
a neutral position (see Figure 6.4).

Avoid sleeping on your stomach with your head turned to one side,
and do not lie on the side where you are experiencing symptoms.
Your best bet is probably to lie on the unaffected side with one pillow
under your head and another pillow in front of you, in line with your
trunk. Use the second pillow to prop up the affected arm.

Do not place your arm overhead, because this stretches the
brachial plexus and puts direct pressure on the nerves in the axilla
(armpit) when you are lying on your side.

An alternative is to lie on your back with one pillow under your head and another pillow under each shoulder and arm, so that the three pillows form an inverted "U". There are several "cervical" pillows on the market; these support the neck without placing stress on the head or cervical spine.

Sleeping on your stomach presents many problems, including the associated arm positions. It is not good for the low back or the neck, so avoid it if possible. If you must sleep on your stomach, try not to use pillows, and keep your arms at your side.

Replace your mattress every ten years, and try several different types before settling on a particular variety. Do not be influenced by claims that mattresses are "orthopedically correct" or doctor approved. The most comfortable type for you is not necessarily the most expensive. If pressure is an issue, a waterbed, especially the waveless type, or a heavily padded mattress can bring relief. These softer beddings tend to conform well to the neck and back.

You might even want to check out adjustable beds, which can increase your choices of sleep positions. For those who have breathing difficulty, a semi-upright posture is very helpful for improving sleep. Adjustable beds can be helpful in this regard. Breathing places significant stress on the trapezial and scalene musculature, so many patients with brachial plexus injury experience increased symptoms during a respiratory infection, because of increased breathing effort, coughing, and sneezing.

7.

Creating a
Comfortable Workplace

Whether or not you realize it, working at a computer takes a toll on your body. Sore muscles, headaches, eyestrain, tension, and fatigue can sometimes result. Fortunately, there is much you can do to help relieve such problems.

Good posture, frequent breaks, stretching exercises, and a comfortable workstation can help keep you from getting stiff, sore, and tired. Exercising at least once an hour–even while sitting at your desk–allows you to release tension that builds up while you work.

In trying to be a productive worker, it's easy to treat computer time as a marathon, but many individuals forget to do the warm-ups and the physical training that can make doing so safe. The habits you develop for making computer work more conducive to your body's needs can be helpful during other activities as well.

YOUR COMPUTER SCREEN, KEYBOARD, AND MOUSE

Sitting in a relaxed, supported position requires arranging your workstation to suit your body. The display should be directly in front of you, at eye height, and adjustable so that you can change it to look up or down for comfort. The key is to avoid straining your neck or arms and to remain comfortable while working.

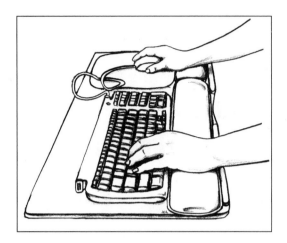

FIGURE 7.1 A Keyboard
and Mouse Wrist Pad Will
Help Properly Align
the Wrists

Laptop computers present two major ergonomic problems: All parts are fixed in position, and people tend to use them in very non-ergonomic postures. Set up your laptop as carefully as you would a desktop computer. Don't put a laptop on top of boxes or use it in awkward sitting postures. Try to use a laptop with a full-sized keyboard and a screen that is easy to read. If your laptop is your full-time computer, set it up ergonomically and attach a full-size mouse and keyboard on a lowered tray with a wrist rest.

As you type or use a mouse, your wrists should be straight, resting in neutral posture using arm rests and/or a wrist rest (see Figure 7.1). This position helps keep pressure off the muscles, tendons, and nerves in the wrists and hands. Prolonged flexing or extending of the wrists can put extra strain on the median nerve in the carpal tunnel. Wrist rests are very helpful for keeping the wrists in proper position and keeping direct pressure off the median and ulnar nerves at the wrist and forearm. It's also important to touch your keys gently, with as little pressure as necessary.

Among various "ergonomic" keyboards available, some work well for some people, but good common sense and proper ergonomics are even more important. Some keyboards simply place the arms and wrists in different abnormal postures, thereby stressing other parts of the arms. My recommendation for any of these alternative appliances is to try it out for at least a half an hour before you purchase it. If it feels good, then it may be helpful, but nothing works for everyone.

The computer mouse is often more of a nemesis than is the keyboard. Reaching to grasp the mouse and holding the wrist up in an extended position for prolonged periods of time frequently lead to repetitive strain and arm injury. If you use a mouse, place it in a position that requires minimal stretch of the arm. If your work requires frequent use of a mouse, consider keeping it on a lowered tray, at the same height as the keyboard, or on your lap. Choose a mouse that fits your hand comfortably and does not require you to posture your hand and wrist abnormally. Better yet, consider the use of a touch pad or voice-activated (recognition) software instead of a mouse and keyboard.

YOUR CHAIR

Chair design is so critical to comfort and health that it is amazing how few chairs are adjustable and suited to the body's ergonomic needs. The seat of the chair at your desk or computer should be firm but not hard. When you are sitting all the way back, your knees should stick out a few inches in front of the seat. Generally speaking, your knees and hips should be at 90-degree angles. The height, back support position, forward tilt, and back tilt of your chair should all be adjustable.

For computer work, the backrest should support your spine when you are sitting up straight. Using a chair that gives way when you sit back produces a tendency to crane the neck forward. A properly adjusted backrest reduces pressure on your spine and supports your lower back. Adjust your backrest until it fits snugly against your lower back. If your backrest is not adjustable, try placing a small pillow or a rolled-up towel at the hollow of your lower back It should feel comfortable; you should not feel as if you are being forced forward in your chair.

ARMRESTS

Armrests help support the shoulders, allowing you to relax the muscles around the neck. They should be short enough to let you come close to your desk, keyboard, or mouse, and adjustable so that you do not have to slouch or hunch your shoulders to reach them (see Figure 7.2). Padded armrests are a good idea if you have nerve problems. Some chairs have removable armrests. For thin or petite people, the armrests are often too far apart to be useful. If you prefer to, or must, work without armrests, be careful not to let your arms hang unsupported while using a keyboard or mouse, because that puts undue strain on the upper arm and neck musculature.

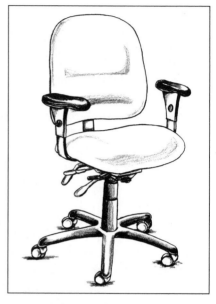

To find your optimal arm position, place your fingers on the middle row of your keyboard and place one hand on the mouse in ready position, with your upper arms relaxed comfortably at your sides. In this position, your fore-

FIGURE 7.2   A Six-Way Adjustable Chair with Armrests Decreases Stress on the Arms, Wrists, and Neck

arms should be parallel to the floor and your wrists resting comfortably in neutral posture. If they are not, adjust your chair height up or down until your forearms are horizontal. If you do not use arm rests, use a padded or gel-type wrist rest to support the weight of your arms. Do the same if you are using a laptop.

Break up tasks and activities to give your arms a rest. If at all possible, schedule activities so that you can take frequent breaks.

FOOT POSITION

Place your feet comfortably in front of you so that your knees bend at a 90-degree angle. Your feet should rest firmly on the floor with three to six inches of leg room between your lap and the keyboard tray (see Figure 7.3). If you can't adjust your desk and chair height so that your feet rest comfortably on the floor, support your feet with a footrest such as a telephone book, or with a wedge-shaped item, such as a

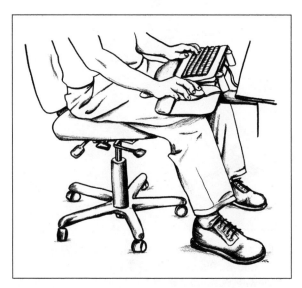

FIGURE 7.3   Feet Should Rest Firmly on the
Floor, with Room to Stretch at Regular Intervals

three-ring binder. Commercially made foot supports and wedges are available as well. You should also have enough room in front of your feet to stretch your legs regularly while working.

WORKSTATION PROPS

Arrange your props so that those you use the most are easily within reach and those you use least often are further away. Your screen or monitor should be straight in front of you, with the top of the monitor at eye height. Place your document holder at the same height and distance as your screen, as much in front of you as possible (see Figure 7.4). Looking off to the left or right while keying puts undue stress on the neck and brachial plexus.

If you are on the phone for regular periods of time, **a headset is a must!** This is one of the simplest ways to avoid neck problems and the most frequently overlooked, both at the office and at home. It is especially vital for those who do other tasks while talking, such as loading the dishwasher or keying at a computer.

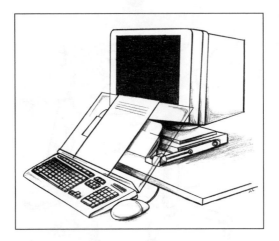

FIGURE 7.4   Props and Computer Screen
Should Be Placed so That They Are Easily
Viewed Without Eye or Neck Strain

Glare is light reflection on your screen, which makes it harder to see the screen clearly. Simple lighting adjustments can help you minimize glare and reduce eye strain. For example, you may move your lamp from behind you to the side to minimize reflection on the screen (see Figures 7.5 and 7.6). Sit in proper working position to check whether your screen is free of glare from sunlight. If you can't adjust window coverings, try turning your display so that it is at a right angle to the window or out of the direct path of harsh lighting, and adjust your desk, keyboard, and chair accordingly.

Adjusting your screen's contrast and brightness can also help

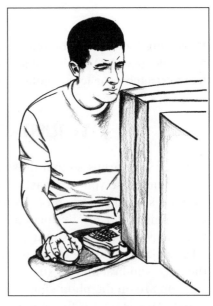

FIGURE 7.5   Glare Can Cause Eye
Strain and Posture Problems

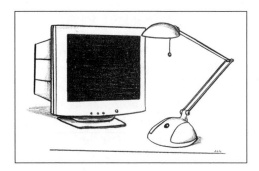

FIGURE 7.6   Good Task
Lighting Is Essential to
Prevent Eye and Neck Strain

improve viewing comfort. Color monitors are better than black-and-white for minimizing eye strain. Some people find anti-glare screen covers helpful.

LIFESTYLE CHANGES

Improving your diet and exercise routine will help you feel better and have more energy. A good exercise routine improves circulation and your body's ability to tolerate the stresses of chronic posturing (sitting in one position for prolonged periods of time) and reaching activity.

Adopting appropriate and correct postures and positions during exercise and other activities helps protect the nerves and minimize tension and undue stress on them.

Rest is also important because it allows time to calm irritation and inflammation around the tissues and nerves.

Each individual has his or her own individual nutritional needs, both personal and physiologic. Two texts I have found to be informative and responsible on these subjects are those by Andrew Weil, M.D., and by Barry Sears, Ph.D., listed in the Bibliography at the back of this book.

Pacing yourself as you work means more than just taking breaks. It involves tackling an appropriate amount of work each day and taking time out between sessions that demand intensive use of the hands and the mind. *Take time to stand and stretch while talking on the telephone or waiting for material to download on your computer.* Breathe deeply, from your belly. Do neck stretches frequently. When you don't need to be looking at the screen, try looking out the window, or close your eyes and relax.

Do not allow yourself to work to the point of pain. Try to take a break even before you feel any early signs of tension or discomfort. Learn to recognize your own personal signals that define your time limits for any given type of task or routine. Take breaks as often as needed, and take them well before you begin to feel fatigue, soreness, or tingling. Symptoms you feel while working are your body's way of telling you that you are doing damage to your soft tissues.

Use pain and discomfort as your guides. They are your friends, and it is prudent to heed their advice.

WORKING WITH TOOLS

Whether you are typing on a computer, working with a jackhammer, or doing light household chores, choose well-designed tools and learn how to modify the way you use your wrists and arms to avoid damage. By not bending, twisting, or extending the wrist, neck, and arms over long periods of time, you can keep extra pressure off your wrists and hands.

If you need to use power tools, look for models with the least possible amount of vibration. Also take steps to minimize exposure to vibration. For example, gloves with extra padding in the palm reduce direct vibration and impact on the median nerve at the hand and wrist.

Alter tools or equipment if necessary, when possible. For example, you might bend a tool or its handle so that you can use it without bending your wrist. Ergonomic hammers are available with pre-bent handles. Consider rotating a tool so that you can hold it with your wrist straight or neutral. Photo 7.1 shows an assortment of ergonomic tools.

In jobs or tasks requiring prolonged and excessive muscle contractions, such as gripping, try not to exert more than a quarter of your maximum force. The more force you exert, the more stress to the nerves and soft tissues. Particularly when using a tool in a repetitive manner or for a prolonged period, try to use as much of your hand as possible when gripping, and avoid pinching with your fingers. Use

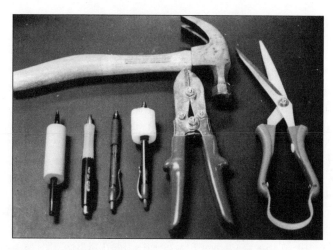

PHOTO 7.1 Ergonomic tools such as these make work easier and put less strain on the hand and arm.

trigger levers (modified devices to activate a tool) rather than single finger press buttons. Alternate hands when possible.

Aggressive gripping stresses the nerve and tendons at the carpal tunnel, causing damage to the nerve and its surrounding tissues, especially if done repetitively.

Studies have documented that simply keeping the wrist in an extended or flexed position, or maintaining sustained grip, increases the pressure in the carpal tunnel, resulting in changes in circulation to the median nerve as well as soft tissue injury.

Prying with a wooden 2-by-4 may seem like a good idea, but when it snaps, you may suffer injury. Separating frozen hamburgers with a sharp knife is a classic mechanism for hand and finger lacerations resulting in nerve and tendon damage. Such injuries are called *accidents* for a reason.

Working with defective equipment is often as dangerous as using the wrong tool. I grimace each time I watch a checker in a store repeatedly rescan an item on a scanning machine that is not reading the bar code correctly. Such repeated strain on the wrist and arm is a sure way to develop a repetitive strain injury. Even scanning repeatedly with a properly functioning scanner can result in repetitive strain injury.

LIFTING AND CARRYING

When standing in good posture, take note of where your hands fall in relation to your body. From this point up to shoulder height is your comfort zone for lifting boxes and working with tools. Try to keep your arms within this region. Avoid reaching above shoulder level or behind your body, because this stresses the brachial plexus.

When lifting an object within your comfort zone, bring the object close to your body and bend your elbows to keep it close (Figure 7.7). This helps limit the amount of force you need to use, thus minimizing weight and pressure on your shoulders. Have a firm footing and a wide stance. When possible, lift one item at a time. You're less likely to strain your muscles if you limit the amount of weight you lift. Bend your knees to go down to the load and keep your back straight. This

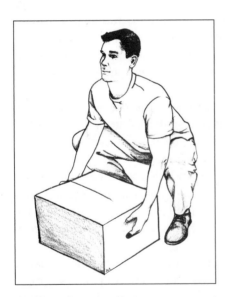

FIGURE 7.7   Use Proper Lifting Techniques at All Times

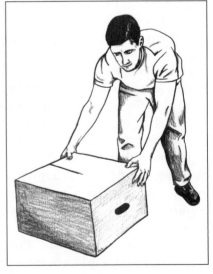

FIGURE 7.8   Do Not Lift While Reaching Away from Your Body, Which Puts Strain on Your Neck and Back

allows you to use the large muscles in your legs designed for heavy activity and minimizes the strain on your back

Avoid reaching too far out from the body (see Figure 7.8). Overhead reaches can put tremendous stress on your neck and brachial plexus. Lifting the arms above shoulder level to support a load tends to increase symptoms of thoracic outlet syndrome. Lean back to stay in balance if necessary and lift the load by straightening the knees. Make it a steady lift. Avoid jerking.

OVERUSE

An important but frequently overlooked issue in patients with an injured extremity is overuse of the uninjured side to compensate for the affected side. Many patients with an initial injury to one arm are not able to perform their usual daily activities, but they try to continue as if there were no problem. Sometimes it is their choice and other times it's a decision forced upon them by an employer, peer pressure, or an insurance carrier. They may attempt to continue two-armed activities using only one arm, often in an awkward and highly inefficient manner. The result is an overuse or abnormal use syndrome in the opposite extremity, which can evolve into a serious disability. In many cases, appropriate rest and decreased demand on the individual as a body early on may avoid long-term permanent injury.

BE YOUR OWN ADVOCATE

At first it might seem that your boss would not agree to the modifications you want for your workstation, chair, computer, or tools. Ask, and you may be pleasantly surprised. Some companies are even proactive and have ergonomics programs in place, evaluating all workstations to optimize design for specific tasks *before* problems develop.

Admittedly, there are many workplaces where employees are afraid to request changes or assistance because they are legitimately afraid that they might lose their job. Your employer needs to appreciate the fact that properly designed equipment will minimize lost work hours and workers' compensation costs, as well as reduce the amount of pain and suffering to injured workers. This is a win-win situation for the employee and the company.

The Americans with Disabilities Act (ADA) is a Federal law that requires employers with fifty or more employees to accommodate injured employees by modifying work spaces or duties so long as the accommodations are reasonable and the employee can perform the essential function of his or her job. Many state laws are enforced by human relations commissions or equal opportunity commissions. Civil Rights sections of state governments have similar laws governing smaller businesses.

For more information, consult your employer, an attorney, or the Equal Employment Opportunity Commission (EEOC) in your region. The Occupational Health and Safety Administration (OSHA) may also be helpful. On the Internet check out www.usdoj.gov/crt/ada/ada-homl/htm, the U.S. Department of Justice ADA home page. *Ability* magazine is another valuable online resource: www.abilitymagazine.com.

In addition to asserting your legal rights, you may want to appeal to your workers compensation carrier, vocational rehabilitation nurse, or medical specialist to intercede or advocate on your behalf. You might tell them, for example, that you can go back to your job if you can get a telephone headset and a better keyboard tray. These items might cost $95, compared to $450 per week for workers compensation, and they could allow the company to retain a valuable employee.

Healing involves taking control of your environment, which often includes advocating for a less harmful workplace.

8.

Effective Splints and
How to Use Them

A splint is an orthopedic device for immobilization, restraint, or support of part of the body. It may be either prefabricated or custom fit. A rigid splint may be made of metal, plaster, or wood. A flexible splint may be made of felt, leather, or a variety of semirigid materials.

Splints are used for a variety of conditions, ranging from fractures, sprains, and nerve injuries to more complex injuries and postoperative care. For example, a patient who has had a severe injury requiring repair of nerves, tendons, and blood vessels could be placed in a dynamic splint. This complex device, made of plastic, metal wires, and elastic bands, gives rigid support to some structures while allowing guided motion in others.

Consumers often purchase prefabricated splints for self-treatment from a pharmacy or medical supply store. Poor design or improper fit can be a problem with these splints, however, and they can lead to further damage by rubbing or irritating the area and putting pressure on already damaged tissues.

The most common prefabricated splint is a wrist brace with a metal support. It can be effective for some people, but for others it can exacerbate carpal tunnel symptoms by holding the wrist tilted up in too much extension, which increases pressure in the carpal tunnel. A splint that hoids the wrist flexed downward can also exacerbate symptoms.

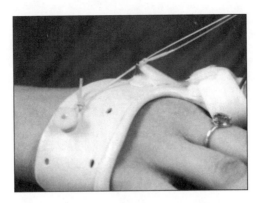

Splints may be customized to accommodate many problems. Such is the case with
this individual, who has an isolated tendon injury to the index finger.

Flexible or semirigid splints help to avoid abnormal use problems
that can occur. Wearing a rigid splint on the wrist results in increased
or abnormal use of other parts of the arm, causing second or even
third levels of nerve involvement (repetitive strain and cumulative
traumas).

The use of custom fabricated splints, designed by physician and
therapist to meet the individual patient's needs, allows optimal positioning to treat the specific injury and fit the individual's anatomy and
physiology. Custom splinting is somewhat more costly but helps
avoid long-term complications that can result from inadequate support, discomfort, and ineffectual results. An inappropriate or uncomfortable splint can be worse than no splint at all.

The appropriate choice of splint for a particular patient depends on
the purpose of the splint, the activities for which it will be used, how
often it will be worn, and whether the splint is for specific activities or
for full-time use. Custom-fit splints may be adjusted for proper fit, to
relieve a point of pressure, or if the patient frequently has swelling
that compromises the fit.

For some types of upper extremity problems, splinting is best done
at the elbow rather than the wrist. For example, if the wrist is splinted
for an individual with an ulnar nerve problem at the elbow, the splint
could cause overuse of the elbow.

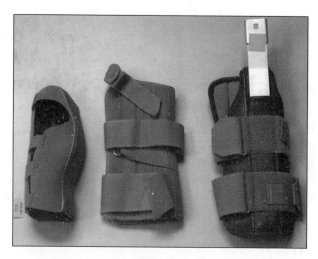

Store-bought splints such as these are sometimes
helpful, but they often put the wrist in the wrong
position and are too rigid to wear during many
activities. (Note the rigid metal bar.)

Wrist splints are appropriate for carpal tunnel nerve injury and tendinitis at the wrist, wrist sprains, stable fractures, ganglion cysts, and
arthritis.

In the acute phase of tendinitis, carpal tunnel symptoms can often
be treated simply by the use of a splint at night. Custom-made rigid
splints are generally the best choice for nighttime use, especially for
nerve problems such as carpal tunnel and tendinitis. By calming the
inflammation associated with the tendinitis, the splint gives relief
from the pressure on the nerve and often reverses the inflammatory
state, essentially making the problem go away.

Splints prevent the wrist from falling into patterns of flexion, in
which the wrist is bent to the palm side, causing compression of the
median nerve at the wrist, which is often a source of tingling and
numbness.

Ideally, patients will use a relatively rigid night splint to rest the inflamed area, combined with activity modification during the day and
a flexible support for stress activities. Nighttime treatment is often
overlooked as the perfect opportunity to rest an injured part with no
inconvenience to the patient.

Custom-made rigid wrist splints are fabricated with a thermoplastic material available from several manufacturers. The therapist makes a pattern of the patient's wrist, then heats the splint in a warm water bath of about 150 degrees F. When the material becomes pliable, the splint is custom molded on the patient. Careful attention is crucial to ensure that the splint fits well so that it does not cause any unnecessary discomfort. Thorough patient education is important for appropriate use.

For support during daytime activities, a semiflexible custom-fabricated splint is the best alternative, because a rigid splint forces the user to compensate, using the upper arm abnormally. Be wary of neoprene splints. They do not give adequate support, and their main source of comfort may be heat retention.

Semiflexible splints made of a combination of athletic training tape, Velcro straps, and felt are very good for daytime use in that they allow motion but still retain relatively neutral posturing of the wrist. Remember,

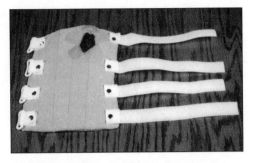

Soft semirigid splints such as this may be worn during activities and at night. Note the absence of a rigid bar in this type of custom splint.

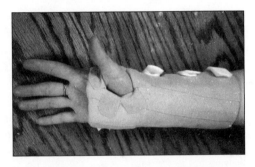

Another semirigid custom splint shown on a patient.

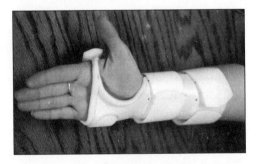

A custom-fabricated wrist splint like this helps decrease swelling when worn at night. Note the wrist is in a neutral position.

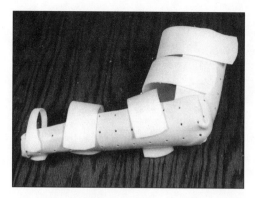

A long arm elbow splint such as this may help patients with ulnar nerve injury at the elbow. It should be worn at night.

daytime use of rigid splints, especially when used to continue repetitive work activities, is dangerous, often worsening an injury.

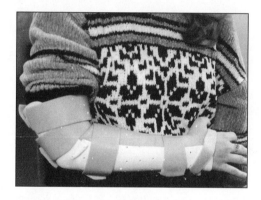

A patient models the long arm elbow splint.

9.

Meditation, Biofeedback, Yoga, and Tai Chi

In addition to maintaining a regular therapy program, it is essential that you incorporate relaxation and stress reduction techniques into your lifestyle. It is often easier to become stressed and dysfunctional than to find truly effective ways to relax. We in fact live in a society that thrives on stress, and its medical implications in causing disease are well documented. Few of us have been taught how to relax or to limit stress throughout the day.

I recognized this fact in painful detail when working with a patient who had a repetitive strain disorder combined with an overstrained voice from using voice-activated software. Severe symptoms prevented him from continuing to work with computers.

When we discussed relaxation and breathing techniques, he told me he understood these and had been doing them for years. I asked him to demonstrate. He took the shallowest breath I have ever seen anyone take when showing me his inhalation technique. His exhalation was equally weak. When he said he had learned his techniques from a book, I realized that personal guidance is often necessary for learning relaxation techniques properly.

Each of us has our own intuitive way of slowing down and relaxing, but regular use of at least one type of relaxation technique is essential for healing and for overall well being. Disciplines such as biofeedback, transcendental meditation, yoga, and tai chi all focus on deep breathing and posture, and all help you decrease the stresses of daily life. Your choice of discipline depends on personal preference, availability of a teacher who suits you, and cost considerations.

Different treatments work best for different patients, so it helps to have a number of options. For example, someone who finds it hard to sit still may benefit more from, say, tai chi or a water-exercise program than from meditation.

Whatever relaxation technique you use, it should help to clear your mind temporarily of outside thoughts and stresses and allow you to focus strictly on what you are doing at the moment. You should expect to complete a session in a relaxed state, usually with your muscles and nerves feeling better.

Many patients find that even if they can only control their pain temporarily in the beginning, at least they realize that it can go away. It gives them a sense of control over something that had previously seemed to control them.

MEDITATION

Meditation, prayer, and focused concentration for healing are age-old and time-tested forms of self healing, recognized by many scientists and philosophers. To quote seventeenth-century philosopher and mathematician Blaise Pascal, "All man's miseries derive from not being able to sit quietly in a room alone." This may be an exaggeration, but the fact is that meditation and relaxation do allow healing of the body and stress relief for the injured organism and its parts.

The common denominator of all meditation techniques is finding a comfortable position; breathing in a relaxed, controlled, and deep manner; and clearing the mind of external thoughts and worries. This allows the body to relax and focus its energy on healing.

Dr. Herbert Benson, one of the first Western doctors to research the use of biofeedback and relaxation techniques to control disease, showed through his work in *The Relaxation Response* (see Bibliography) that definite long-term physiologic and psychological advantages occurred when ordinary people practiced meditation techniques twice daily for twenty minutes at a time. The changes included control and lowering of high-blood pressure and an overall improved sense of well being. Further, Dr. Benson found that when the practice stopped, the beneficial effects of the techniques disappeared. The type of meditation did not matter; be it yoga, transcendental meditation, or another form of deep breathing, the most important element was regular, continued practice.

Meditation techniques often allow patients with nerve pain and injury to better deal with pain and decrease its intensity. As stress decreases, muscle spasms decrease, which lessens the direct pressure on the nerves and improves their blood supply.

BIOFEEDBACK

Biofeedback uses a machine to tell you how much you are relaxing while performing deep-breathing exercises. Most patients need about twelve sessions to learn the technique with a qualified biofeedback therapist or psychologist. Once learned, it is important to continue practicing biofeedback. Many people use a tape-recorded program to gain practice experience, which increases the effectiveness of the technique.

It is important that the therapist understand your specific individual needs and which muscles you especially want to relax. For thoracic outlet syndrome, repetitive strain injury, fibromyalgia, or significant neck injury, it is important to relax the scalene muscles and the upper trapezial area. Biofeedback, when performed appropriately, should provide increased blood flow to the arms, which increases circulation to the intrinsic blood supply of the nerves. This allows softening of the scar tissue that surrounds the injured nerves, which allows further healing.

Meditation alone without biofeedback hookup can achieve similar effects, but it helps to have a "feedback" mechanism, at least initially, so that you can see how well you are doing.

YOGA AND TAI CHI

Yoga and tai chi are both excellent means for reducing stress and stretching the muscles and neurovascular structures. Some people think of tai chi as meditation in motion. Its smooth, slow motions allow nerve sliding along with the benefits of deep breathing.

Both yoga and tai chi are meant to be done gently and slowly. Look for a well-qualified teacher who understands your nerve problem. Once you learn the basic techniques, you may have enough discipline to practice at home without a teacher; however, continued work with a teacher can result in much greater benefits, increasing over years of practice. I recommend at least an initial six sessions to learn some basic techniques to perform at home.

ALTERNATIVE AND COMPLEMENTARY TREATMENTS

Many patients have found relief from acupuncture, chiropractic and osteopathic manipulation, reflexology, massage, deep muscle therapy, craniosacral therapy, or other complementary or integrative therapies, used either with or without other forms of treatment. There is no single best approach for all patients or all conditions. If one treatment does not help, keep searching until you find what works for you. Search among different practitioners within a given treatment approach in addition to considering different types of treatment. Success often depends upon finding the right person. None of these treatments should be painful. Pain is your body's way of telling you that something is wrong and that it is time to try a different approach.

Unlike many of today's exercise and therapy programs that overstress and overstretch us, meditation and relaxation techniques are lifetime pursuits. They allow slow, steady progress with no pain and all gain.

10.

A Home-Based Exercise
and Healing Program

The key to any exercise program is to be sure that it feels good. Although you might feel fatigued after you exercise, you should not have any pain or discomfort from strained joints, ligaments, or tendons. Nerve pain is not an acceptable by-product of an exercise program.

Exercise needs often change once you reach your thirties or early forties, have an injury, or have long-term disabilities. Various stresses and responsibilities in our lives–and shifting priorities–change the overall activity level of our daily routines in a sedentary society. Exercise and "free time" give way to the needs of our finances and family responsibilities. Growing out of shape is not as much an aging process as it is a fact of life in a high-paced and stressed society. For many, exercise becomes an obligation rather than a desire. This is a fact for many of us, with and without injury.

Because of the relatively poor conditioning that most of us achieve, warming up before exercise, cooling down afterward, and extensive stretching become increasingly vital with age and injury.

Exercise is essential in any healing and treatment program. Its proven benefits include the body's release of endorphins and enkephalins via pituitary action; these help to decrease pain and dysfunction and produce emotional and physical feelings of well being. In fact, the strength of these natural pain killers is much more powerful than any known human-made narcotic.

The type of exercise you choose matters less than making exercise a regular routine. Whether you have heart disease, fibromyalgia, arthritis, musculoskeletal disorders, or nerve pain, routine exercise will change the way your body deals with disease processes and how it heals.

Regular walking, both outdoors and indoors on a treadmill, is a great form of exercise. If you have arm or wrist symptoms, limit arm swings by sticking your hands in pockets.

Exercises in water can be particularly helpful, especially for patients who do not tolerate the pressures of gravity and the stresses of their own body weight or the weight of their arms. Pool exercise can range from a modified aerobics program to simply walking about in the water. Remember to avoid motions and activities that result in discomfort or increased symptoms.

Tai chi, yoga, and other traditionally Eastern forms of exercise have underlying beneficial effects of internal aerobic conditioning, muscle toning, and strengthening. Through the benefits of deep breathing and gentle strengthening of the intercostal, diaphragmatic, and upper trapezial musculature, tai chi and yoga exercises are quite helpful in stabilizing many upper extremity nerve problems. The aerobic and metabolic effect of these exercises is much more subtle, but the sweat and benefit can approach more active, traditionally Western forms of working out. They ideally should be combined with a true aerobic program such as swimming or walking, if medically tolerated, for optimal results.

The actual motions incorporated in these types of exercise are quite beneficial to nerve entrapment. In fact, many are similar to the postures and movements used in the nerve sliding techniques described in Chapter 4.

Sam, a patient of mine with a passion for trout fishing, once described to me the way he holds the rod and reel and moves the line out and away from his body. The motions are slow and rhythmic, and when Sam observed himself in this relatively meditative state of bliss doing his fishing, he noted that the posture and movements were the same as the nerve sliding exercises we had taught him. He realized that, in fact, he felt no pain during salmon fishing tournaments, which last for up to eight hours.

When you evaluate any type of exercise program, look at those who have been doing it for many years. Do they continue to tolerate the program into their sixties, seventies, eighties, and even nineties? If so, this may be a good exercise program for you!

Within a given form of exercise, one style may be more appropriate than another for the long term. For example, compare various styles of the martial arts. Some are based more on softness and the ability to move and avoid injury by deflecting and redirecting blows and assaults. Other styles are based on the concept of aggressive strength training, which promotes the theory that strength allows a person to absorb blows and hit back with great power. The idea is to meet force with force, which makes both opponents vulnerable to injury. Much of Chinese medicine evolved from efforts by martial arts practitioners to treat the injuries they inflicted upon each other.

The softer approach is based on deflecting force and avoiding injury. Similarly, you should look for exercise forms that do not injure your body.

Weight training on a limited basis with light weights may be useful for strengthening once pain is gone, but it has been our experience that using weights aggressively increases muscle bulk and adds significant undue stress on the nervous system. We have not found great benefits to aggressive weight training and in many cases have found that it is harmful to individuals with upper extremity disorders.

This applies to common sense at home as well. Recently my wife and I were walking in a park. A fragile woman, who was around seventy years old, was walking in front of us, obviously for exercise. This was commendable, except she was carrying heavy weights in her hands, which pulled her so far forward that her knuckles were just about dragging on the ground. Her good efforts would no doubt be met with a stronger heart, but very soon she would be bound to experience significant neck and arm pain. Her friends and doctor told her that weights were good for her osteoporosis, but in fact this was an unhealthy approach.

Judicious use of light weights may be helpful for some medical conditions such as osteoporosis, but the benefits must be gained without damaging other parts of your body. "Water walking," with the water as the weight and resistance, would serve many people–including the woman we saw in the park–better and be gentler on the nerves.

If your desire is to maintain muscle tone and strength, then I recommend simply doing push-ups, sit-ups, and leg lifts.

Push-ups should first be performed by standing and pushing away from a wall. Start close to the wall and gradually increase your distance. Once you are comfortable, start using the back of a chair, then use the seat of a chair.

When you are secure and comfortable with this, move to floor push-ups. Begin from a kneeling position and graduate to full push-ups on your toes, with the knees off the ground.

Try not to do push-ups on your palms. This puts tremendous stress on the wrists and carpal tunnel. Do them on your knuckles, on a soft rug. Or try a stand that allows you to grip, keeping the wrists straight; these are available in athletic specialty stores.

Eventually you may be able to do push-ups on your fingertips, which strengthens the forearms as well as the flexor and extensor tendon muscles, helping to stabilize the wrists and tone the upper body. As with any athletic activity, when performing these exercises, use a spotter or coach to protect you and help prevent injury.

Sit-ups and leg lifts not only tone the abdominal muscles but also enhance the function of the muscles used for breathing. Place your hands on the back of your head to support your neck and upper back while doing these.

The ideal exercise does not stress or pound on the cartilage in joints, which can cause erosion and long-term changes, including arthritis. The ideal exercise also avoids overstretching and stressing of tendons, ligaments, and nerve structures. However, activity must be aggressive enough to elevate the heart rate and increase circulation to the nerves, vital organs, and other musculoligamentous structures. The goal is to find something enjoyable that will bring about beneficial effects without injury.

11.

How to Set Up Your Own Home Therapy Center

Some patients are capable of setting up a therapy program and unit at home that ends up being as good as, if not better than, many of the therapy units available in formal therapy centers. Tom, who is a machinist, had significant problems with his hands. He had severe carpal tunnel symptoms and a significant repetitive strain injury. He had problems with triggering in his fingers as well as numbness, tingling, and pain.

Tom got some relief from therapy, but as soon as he stopped treatment for more than a week, his symptoms increased.

Unfortunately, during the course of his treatment his health plan cut off his coverage because a doctor who reviewed his case decided that he had received adequate therapy, even though he remained symptomatic. One of the doctors who saw Tom advised his insurance carrier that under no circumstances should Tom ever have surgery, because if he did, he might develop a reflex-sympathetic dystrophy.

This left Tom with the option of either living with his symptoms as they were, with the probability that they would worsen, or having surgery, which his treating doctor recommended but his insurer would not cover. Basically, Tom became a victim of the system, falling outside the norms of the "standard of care" with respect to his injuries. He was therefore cut off from any treatment that would provide relief, and he was also denied the option of surgery.

Tom couldn't afford to pay for surgery, medications, or therapy on his own. He felt he was really between a rock and a hard place.

Using his skills as a machinist, Tom constructed his own home therapy unit. He built a whirlpool and a paraffin dip bath. He also utilized other standard modalities such as a high-voltage unit and deep heating pads (not home assembled). Thus, not only was he able to give himself the therapy he had previously received from our clinic but he could also do it daily, as often as needed. He stabilized his symptoms and made them totally tolerable. Although Tom might have benefited from surgery, he found a way to improve without it!

Few of us are as talented and resourceful as Tom, but the self-help concept is available to anyone who is willing to use a little ingenuity and make use of readily available healing tools. I do not recommend building therapy units on your own unless you are a qualified electrician and machinist, because of the danger of electrical shock. We can, however, with a little thought and incentive achieve success as Tom did.

HOW YOU CAN DEVELOP AN INDIVIDUALIZED, IN-HOME THERAPY PROGRAM

Step one. Assess exactly which types of modalities and treatments have been successful for you. They could include heat or cold treatments, ranging from a hot tub soak or showers to asking your spouse to massage you in a manner that is similar to professional massage treatments. We even have had patients whose spouses come in to learn appropriate massage from our therapists.

Step two. Obtain the appropriate modality units for your home. They can include home hydroculator packs (hot packs), high-voltage units (not home assembled), transcutanous electrical nerve stimulation (TENS) units, or other tools for standard therapy. A sauna or whirlpool can be useful in the home (where it can be enjoyed by the whole family) or at a health club. Massage chairs and portable hand-held units and pads are sometimes helpful, but they can be a bit too aggressive, so be wary.

Try to create an area where you will go for therapy on a regular basis. To incorporate endurance training into your program, you might wish to purchase a low-impact stepper, rower, treadmill, bicycle, or elliptical or cross-trainer type of machine.

Step three. Evaluate your sleeping environment. Is your mattress too hard, too soft, or too old to give you adequate support? Do you have enough pillows? If you have difficulty sleeping comfortably, it might be worth investigating alternative types of mattresses or pillows filled with water, down, or high-tech synthetics.

Step four. Once you have determined which modalities and what type of program would be helpful to you, run the list by your therapist to ensure that you are on the right track with your program and that it is consistent with what has been beneficial to you. Contact your physician as well. Write to your health plan asking for approval and help in setting up your home program. Point out that your approach will result in large cost-savings to the health plan.

Insurers often have ideas on where to get items at discount and will in many cases work with you to obtain the appropriate items. If a local health club has the appropriate facilities or modalities, consider joining the club as part of your plan, especially if it is affordable and conveniently located.

Step five. Be sure to take time in your daily routine to utilize what you have learned. Make appropriate time for biofeedback, meditation, or another relaxation technique in your program. Twenty minutes in the morning and twenty minutes in the evening for relaxation techniques is enough for most people, but some need more time. Be sure there is a "quiet area" where you can do it.

Step six. When doing your therapy, remember that stretching, warming up, and cooling down are essential and that stretches and nerve slides are also imperative. Although you may be using therapy modalities in your program, the stretching and motion portion is as important as–if not more important than–the modalities themselves.

Step seven. Set up a schedule for yourself and follow it. Even if you don't have all the modalities you want or your home is not yet set up, begin treating yourself at home.

Start your home program even when you are in formal therapy, so that you can augment the therapy program. Be careful not to overstrain or overexercise, but once you begin a home program, make it part of your daily life and routine. Others in your family are likely to be supportive, and they might even join in. Sharing in the healing process brings people together and allows a more open understanding of your pain.

A home program helps put you in control of your pain, your healing, and your life. Although you may not be able to cure yourself, very often you can augment and extend the temporary relief you are getting from medical professionals, ultimately gaining the ability to give yourself relief whenever you want it!

Whether it is fibromyalgia, repetitive strain injury, carpal tunnel, thoracic outlet syndrome or another type of pain syndrome, you know your body, your nerves, and your injuries better than anyone else. Although medical practitioners may be able to evaluate and treat you, they are not living in your body. You live every minute of every day with your pain, discomfort, and disability. This gives you a distinct advantage in designing a treatment program. As long as you go slowly and remember that pain and discomfort are your warning signs, you should be able to move ahead with the healing process.

Step eight. Examine your eating habits and schedule. Leave enough time to eat regular and healthy meals. Take time to enjoy food. Your body can only swallow and assimilate a meal in a set amount of time, and if you rush the process, indigestion and increased stress will be counterproductive in the long run. Most people feel better when they develop healthy eating habits and a more regular eating schedule.

Vitamin B and B-complex vitamins are often helpful in nerve healing. Researchers have shown that the antioxidant vitamins C and E aid in tissue healing and help to slow or even reverse the destructive process of oxidation of the tissues in the body. Taking multivitamins daily helps ensure that you do not create any deficiencies.

Researchers are currently trying to confirm the validity of glucosamine and chondroitin sulfate in the treatment of degenerative joint disease and the regeneration of cartilage. Many people have had good experience with this, but the findings are not yet based on strict clinical studies.

12.

A Final Thought

There are many ways that we as patients can treat ourselves at home without having to go to a doctor or use a therapy unit. I get e-mail from people all around the world asking how they can obtain treatment when none of the doctors or therapists available to them are familiar with their particular nerve problems. I tell them that the key to healing is to have an understanding of your own disease. Once you understand the basic anatomy, physiology, and mechanism through which your disease happens, therapy visits can be as necessary or unnecessary as doctor visits. Once you have a program and a good idea of what needs to be done, self-treatment is often the answer.

Simple modalities that you can use in your own home include your shower and bathtub (I especially like long tub soaks to relieve multiple body aches). Many people use Epsom salts in the bath for a soothing effect. Pulse showerheads are also quite good for hydromassage.

Other simple modalities include heating pads, sunshine, and avoiding cold drafts.

A local YMCA or health club with a spa, whirlpool, or sauna is certainly a good place to obtain deep heat. Many of our patients have hot tubs and whirlpools in their homes and use them once or twice a day. This is greatly helpful for mobilizing not only the affected areas but also the entire body. It also improves the ability to perform stretching exercises and relaxation techniques. Home paraffin units are another excellent form of deep heat. Warm soaks for hand and arm, as well as for feet problems, are also beneficial.

Once you learn basic stretching exercises, be sure to continue doing the stretches and slides regularly. Maintaining flexible and supple tissues makes them less prone to repeated and new injury. Furthermore, when joints and ligaments are stretched regularly, they hurt less and your function, circulation, and healing potential all improve.

Muscles, ligaments, and tendon structures should be gently and progressively stretched. Expect to gain increased flexibility or motion not in one or two sessions but rather over the course of weeks and months. Once you achieve more flexibility, you just need to maintain it first thing in the morning and in the evening before going to bed.

Limitations on the type of exercise one should incorporate are only bound by the imagination. Exercise should be modified to suit your own style and physical capabilities and limitations. The key is to do something on a regular basis so that you continue to move.

There is no doubt that many patients who suffer from repetitive strain injury, carpal tunnel injury, fibromyalgia, and nerve pain can be treated and get better without surgery, and many others can get better with limited surgery and medication. People heal by understanding how their disease has affected their lives and changing to a healthier lifestyle.

These thoughts are not solely those of one physician. Many of us in the medical community have come to realize that we need to start trusting our patients more by allowing them to use their own innate abilities to heal.

My philosophy for wellness is fairly simple. Set a goal. Make a plan to get to that goal. The plan should be realistic and within your physical capabilities. Physicians and therapists can help by increasing awareness of necessary behavior and lifestyle changes, but only you know where you want to be and how to get there.

Writing down goals has proven helpful for many of our patients. I often recommend writing goals in sequential plans. Here is an exercise for you to try:

On one sheet of paper, write down where you want your life to be six months, one year, five years, and ten years from now. Address all aspects of your life, including marriage, travel, career, schooling, finances, friends, retirement, and anything else you may be concerned about.

The moment you write something down, it becomes more than a passing thought. It becomes part of your reality. Once you stop mulling over the same thoughts over in your head time after time and actually see your own ideas on paper, things start to happen. If you review and revise your list every day, you begin to formulate plans and ways to turn your ideas into reality.

Remember, nothing in this world ever happened until it was originally a thought or a dream in someone's mind. The automobile, the airplane, landing a man on the moon, all began as thoughts and fantasies in someone's mind. Once the idea exists, the creation of reality ensues. When you consider that humans utilize less than 10 percent of their brain's potential, it is easy to conceive that self-healing through a plan is easily achievable.

The above is simply a template for you to follow with respect to a healing program. Each individual will require his or her own program, and every person will do it differently. The key is simply *to do it*, and take your healing and health into your own hands.

I thank you, the reader, for taking the time to review and understand this information. I also thank patients for taking the bold step of being proactive in their own care. For readers who are medical practitioners in the healing arts, I thank you for taking care of your patients so as to avoid injury rather than attempting to treat it after the fact, especially with surgery, which in many cases is not successful.

I wish each reader the best of health and success without surgery.

Appendix:
Resources for
Home Therapy Centers

Ameriphone, Inc.
800-874-3005
E-mail: meriphone@ameriphone.com
Web site: www.ameriphone.com
Manufactures assistive telecommunication devices. Products include remote-controlled voice-activated speakerphones, amplified telephones, and telephone accessories.

Amrex Electrotherapy Equipment
800-221-9069
E-mail: amrex@amrex-zetron.com
Web site: www.amrex-zetron.com
A manufacturer of electrotherapy equipment for more than sixty years. The Amrex line includes ultrasound, electrical stimulation devices, and TENS.

AquaTrend, Inc.
800-296-5496
E-mail: info@aquatrend.net
Web site: www.aquatrend.net
Manufactures and distributes aquatic exercise and rehab equipment for professional and home use.

BioMedical Life Systems, Inc.
800-726-8367
E-mail: information@bmls.com
Web site: www.bmls.com
Manufactures electromedical devices and accessories such as high-volt pulsed stimulators, TENS, and a complete line of electrodes.

Body Therapeutics
909-674-5722
E-mail: btwilhelm@juno.com
Manufactures various support pillows, back supports, and cervical and lumbar rolls.

Chess Publications
800-467-5943
Publishes health care books for the general public.

Comfort Keyboard Systems Co., Inc.
414-481-2056
E-mail: cksystems@aol.com
Web site: www.comfortkeyboard.com
Manufacturers ergonomic keyboards and other ergonomic devices for the workplace or home office.

J and J Medical
800-494-8680
Web site:
Provides electrical stimulation equipment and a large variety of health care supplies.

Bibliography and Suggested Reading

Benson, Herbert. *The Relaxation Response.* New York: Avon Books, 1970.

——. *Beyond the Relaxation Response: How to Harness the Healing Power of Your Personal Beliefs.* New York: Times Books, 1984.

Dyer, Wayne. *Your Erroneous Zones.* New York: HarperPerennial, 1991.

Fried, Scott. *Light at the End of the Carpal Tunnel: A Guide to Understanding and Relief from the Pain of Nerve Problems.* East Norriton, PA: Healing Books, 1998.

Hill, Napoleon. *Think and Grow Rich.* Hollywood, FL: Lifetime Books, 1998.

Hunter, James, Evelyn Mackin, and Ann Callahan. *Rehabilitation of the Hand: Surgery and Therapy.* 4th ed. St. Louis, MO: Mosby-Yearbook, 1995.

Kabat-Zinn, Jon. *Full Catastrophe Living: Using the Wisdom of Your Body and Mind to Face Stress, Pain, and Illness.* New York: Bantam Doubleday Dell Publishing Group, 1991.

Saunders, Richard. *Thoracic Outlet Syndrome: A Common Sequela of Neck Injuries.*Philadelphia: J. B. Lippincott, 1990.

Sears, Barry. *A Week in the Zone: A Quick Course in the Healthiest Diet for You.* New York: Harper Collins Publishers, 2000.

Siegel, Bernie S. *Love, Medicine, and Miracles: Lessons Learned About Self-Healing from a Surgeon's Experience with Exceptional Patients.* New York: HarperPerennial, 1990.

Weill, Andrew. *Eating Well for Optimum Health.* New York: Random House, 2000.

Index